Come Ride with Me along the Big C

Dear Rossi,

I'm so thrilled that we met at the River! I can't wait to come to your class soon. I hope you enjoy the story!

Love
Claire

Come Ride with Me along the Big C

Printed in the United States of America
ISBN: 978-1497520189

Learn more information at:
www.oceansoulyoga.com

To Todd, for always believing in me.

When the Japanese mend broken objects, they aggrandize the damage by filling the cracks with gold. They believe that when something has suffered damage and has a history it becomes more beautiful.

Barbara Bloom

Chapter 1 January

Friday, January 1: Welcome Twenty-Ten

I feel optimistic, clear and ready to embrace 2010; a year filled with harvesting all the seeds sown in 2009. After more than a decade of vowing to exit corporate America, I finally quit my job forever. The champagne flowed to celebrate that there will be no more practicing law. No more outside sales. No more worrying about quotas and billable hours.

In a dozen years, I had about the same number of careers. When it became apparent that I didn't seem to care much for confrontation, all signs indicated that I may have made a very expensive mistake called law school. Of course, I do miss wearing those short Ally McBeal suits and high heels to court.

To the chagrin and bafflement of many people I knew and more that I didn't, I plunged headfirst into the life of a full time yoga instructor. Finally! Career Number 13 fit. Teaching yoga, Pilates and writing articles on wellness is satisfying beyond belief. And, I'm doing it on a big scale. Not only am I on track to publish articles in national fitness magazines, I'm also collaborating with Exercise TV to film some yoga/Pilates workouts for them and was recently selected as a lululemon ambassador. From attorney to ambassador for a major yoga lifestyle company in one short year: yes!

On a health note, this is Year One after my neck disc-replacement surgery. For the most part, I've felt fantastic but surprise, surprise, I overdid it a few times and suffered from setbacks. Learning to be patient with my

1

limitations is one of my greatest challenges. As patience is not one of my greatest virtues, I've got my work cut out for me. Perhaps I should practice what I preach to my yoga and Pilates students?

Onward and upward.

Friday, January 8th: Mike's Hard Lemonade

Okay, the waking up in the middle of the night is getting old. It is 4:34 a.m. For the sixth night in a row I can't sleep. Why am I suffering from insomnia? On Saturday night, January 2nd, while applying body lotion after taking a shower, I found a lump in my breast. It felt like someone had inserted a marble under my skin. An alien marble. An interloper. It felt absolutely wrong. Immediately, I knew that it was serious.

Sunday crawled at a snails' pace.

On Monday, I saw my doctor, who after examining me, told me that it was most likely nothing. Nonetheless, she scheduled me for a diagnostic mammogram and potential ultrasound for today, Friday. I had to sweat it out for four days. Wondering.

After my mammogram and ultrasound this morning, the doctor entered the room to inform me that she had scheduled me for a biopsy in a few hours. Huh? Fast forward to another sterile room and the biopsy doctor bluntly informed me that the irregular shape of the lump was very worrisome and most likely cancerous. I'm sorry, what? My 2010 vision board clearly indicated that this is my year to regain my health, not the year that I get cancer.

Immediately upon finishing the biopsy, I exited the room, saw my boyfriend Todd, and burst into tears. The doctor

2

had offered me Xanax, but I demurred. All I wanted was to go to the beach and watch the breathtaking sunset and absorb some love from the ocean. It always calms me. But, something told me that I needed more than nature today. I needed a drink. A stiff drink. Not my usual method of handling stress, but in the circumstances, I think it wasn't out of line.

We pulled into the first liquor store we saw, in the charming village of Del Mar, California. As I perused my choices, I realized that a large beer wouldn't do because I'd be full before being able to take the edge off of my news. So, I chose a Mike's Hard Lemonade. In a quart bottle. We dressed it up in a plain paper bag and as my boyfriend Todd drove us through Del Mar, I guzzled it.

Yes, I chugged it out of a brown paper bag. Where are the paparazzi when you need them? What a photo opportunity: me turning down Xanax for some malt liquor. It numbed my mind but couldn't stop the tears from streaming. Watching the sunset with my love also helped. (The "my love" reference is for Todd, not the Mike's Lemonade, in case you were wondering.)

Saturday, January 9th: Day 7 without sleep
Maybe I should have accepted the Xanax? I have to say this has not been the most auspicious beginning to 2010.

Sunday, January 10th:
I don't remember today. At all.

Monday, January 11th:

Today wasn't a bad day waiting for the diagnosis. I taught my Pilates class, kicked my own butt working out in the Pilates studio, taught yoga and chilled in the afternoon. Taught another yoga class and came home and soaked up the always cheesy and entertaining The Bachelor. I offer no apologies-it is about the only show I ever watch and it never fails to amuse. I was asked to be a contestant on it a few years back, but that is another story. I turned that one down as I believe they were setting me up to be the cougar-HA!

Tuesday, January 12th: The Phone Call

8:20 a.m.-As I careened down the highway, running late for my Tuesday morning yoga class, my ringing phone's display indicated Scripps Hospital calling. Picking up the phone, I receive the news that will forever alter my life.

They informed me that the pathology results were positive; there is cancer present. Wow. No details on the stage or size of the tumor. Just cancer. All my questions would be answered on Wednesday at 11:15 a.m. at the Surgery Center. She suggested that I spend time with someone that day as she didn't think I should be alone. Well, no. Probably not.

Immediate dilemma: how the hell was I going to teach my class in 5 minutes? Then I realized that I love my class, I love teaching yoga and I was just going to do it. Todd was in Colorado for a big client presentation and I left him the news on voicemail. Probably not my most considerate move but hey, sometimes selfishness prevails.

Upon arriving at Sculpt Fusion Yoga, I informed Kim, the owner, and she enveloped me in a big hug. One of my favorite students, Helene, also heard and their support felt tangible. Everything flowed in class and it was beautiful.

After class, I chatted a bit and then dove into practice. Teacher Jenn kicked our butts and I spent a good portion of the class in child's pose. But, it had to have been better than not taking class, right? I am writing like a third grader, but that is okay for right now. I will let go of my University of Virginia English major status for present.

After yoga, for some reason, I thought that going to get a manicure/pedicure was the best idea. And, it was. For some reason, grooming really calms me down and perks me up. My friend Kirsten came and joined me: girl time rocks.

Wednesday, January 13th: First Post-diagnosis appointment of a million

At the appointment today, the doctor shared some encouraging news. As of now, the cancer is Stage 1 unless they find evidence it spread. My dance card is filling fast with diagnostic tests. In addition to an MRI, I've got a BSGI scheduled for Tuesday morning. The BSGI should reveal if the pesky cancer cells have swam into other unwelcome areas.

Surgery is definitely on the menu, but not for another few weeks: just lots of fun tests for now. They also don't know yet if it will be lumpectomy and radiation, the "M" word (I seriously hope not) or if chemo will be recommended. No. Don't want that at all. I plan on eating all my spinach and pulling a Popeye on this crap.

The doctors keep reassuring me that if the "M" does happen that they have fabulous plastic surgeons and reconstruction is included...or if it is the lumpectomy, they will tighten and lift it up a bit. I asked if they would also do that for the left one and apparently, you can get a free boob lift out of this. Finally-the silver lining: perky girls until I am 80.

Friday, January 15th: Brain Drain Begins

Today's MRI was my least favorite procedure, well, oops, my second least favorite of the last few weeks. The needle biopsy last week was terrible and I have the black and yellow bruises to prove it. Today, however, I faced the discordant cacophony emanating inside the MRI chamber. Gunfire, jackhammer, 1980's speed-metal; take your pick. When I had an MRI of my neck a few years ago, I was convinced that my brain was being drained by the alien sounding noise. Think The Matrix. An insidious stealing of your brain through the ear.

So, I was prepared for that. Not happy, but nevertheless prepared. Being subjected to this seemingly endless myriad of tests makes me feel like a science experiment. Or, that I've been captured by the above-referenced aliens and they are testing me to see if they'll just dissect me for parts or if I may be worthy for breeding little half-aliens. As you can tell, the MRI's deafening coffin-like interior is not designed for those with a vivid imagination.

My fun began with an IV being inserted into my arm for the purpose of injecting dye into my system. Apparently, the dye reveals irregularities on the MRI. Nobody told me about the IV. Perhaps this would be considered a pertinent tidbit of information for the person to be pierced? I hate needles. In the past, nurses would laugh at me because I had to lie down anytime I gave blood or I would faint. A warning about the ink injection would have been appreciated.

As I am not blessed with a poker face, I could not feign indifference. It hurt. It grossed me out. And, again, it made me feel like a specimen. But, the fun was only beginning. Next, I was told to open my robe and lay face-down, arranging my boobs into two slots and flattening my face into a massage table head-rest. Sadly, this wasn't a massage.

Picture me face down with tennis shoes and socks peeking out from the robe. Arms stretched overhead with the above-referenced unwelcome IV protruding. To complete my ensemble, the technician stuffed a pair of giant headphones from the 1980's onto my head to provide music. Where is a good photographer when you need one? I'm determined to find that silver lining each step of the way. The best I can do here is to appreciate that the first song was Somewhere Around Midnight, one of my favorites. Unfortunately, it couldn't drown out the horrible brain-sucking sounds of the MRI machine.

Test ended. IV removed. Ouch. Red tape wrapped around my bandaged arm. Since my diagnosis, everyone tells me to avoid sugar. That it causes cancer cells to multiply, that it is the breeding ground for everything from the devil to yes, cancer. And, I've been good so far.

Distraught after this fourth invasion in less than a week, I proceeded to the closest bakery. Sporting a large welt across my forehead from the machine, I must have looked more forlorn and pathetic than I realized because the bakery lady allowed me to not only select my cinnamon roll, but she also warmed it up and added extra frosting.

Said cinnamon roll was approximately the size of my head. My head is large. It was the perfect fuel for teaching my 10:35 a.m. yoga class at Frogs Encinitas. I won't have any sugar tomorrow, promise. I don't want to get cancer or anything.

Okay, I'm going to read now. Something unrelated to this disease.

An overwhelming thank you to everyone in my life for the generous outpouring of love and support. I am amazed, humbled, and blessed to have such a powerful circle around me and I need and love each and every one of you.

Saturday, January 16th: Beautiful

Today was exactly what I needed. I went to a yoga workshop with the incredible Erich Schiffman. He was funny, inspiring and made meditation seem simple and natural. He is magical. Sharing the experience with my friends Summer and Renee left e feeling relaxed and positive.

Over the last few weeks, I couldn't help feeling like I am reaping some serious karma. Those who know me are aware that my family has endured great tragedy. I mean, what are the odds that two siblings pass away from AIDS, one dies from other causes and both daughters get breast cancer? My sister beat it with grace and beauty and so will I.

We are like the poor Kennedys, but if you have to deal with this much crap in one family, you should at least have your own yacht. Here's my theory: in a past life we were the Genghis Khans and now it is payback time. All that pillaging, raping, and beheading really takes its toll. The lessons in grief and mourning have been intense, to put it mildly. But, we are a hardy lot. Probably the Corsican blood on my dad's side of the family. Coupled with the Scottish McNeill clan on my mom's side, this lifetime is presenting some hefty challenges.

A very wise woman, who is an artist and astrologer, shared a beautiful perspective with me. Victoria's advice verbatim:

You just have some big Life Long Lessons, like the rest of us, and you are working to balance them out. And you will. Sometimes the "healer" type people, like you, have to become the "wounded healer" for a time, until some kind of energy transmutation takes place. If this is part of some kind of shamanic journey, then so be it, let's just get it over with fast so you can heal and get on with the business of living a beautiful life and helping others. I know that is your destiny.

I do believe the loss I've experienced with my family has made me stronger and more empathetic and better equipped to help others. And, since today is my one year anniversary of exiting corporate America to teach yoga and Pilates full-time, I do feel that I am on my true path to heal and help.

I like it. Although I id believe that the 2007 car accident resulting in an artificial disc replacement in my neck was plenty of wounding. Apparently not?

Monday, January 18th: Not such a good day

Okay, I am cresting the rollercoaster. Immediately upon waking this morning, I sensed it was not going to be one of my energetic, adrenaline filled days. Yesterday was spent consuming an amazing book about Natural Medicine and Cancer. An excellent resource, I liked it because it discusses using both natural/holistic methods in combination with medical treatment. As part of the yoga community, I've received a great deal of well meaning advice about how to treat my cancer without conventional medicine. While I appreciate the intentions, all I can say is that rubbing herbs on my boob, chugging kale shakes and partaking in coffee enemas does not feel like the correct prescription for me. I want the lump out. Excised. No questions asked.

Horrible appointment this morning. Horrible, horrible, horrible. It all began when I went alone to see the Radiation Oncologist. Huge mistake. Now I understand why everyone told me to always bring someone with you to the appointments. Lesson learned.

Dr. Radiation told me that based on the MRI from Friday (remember that visual? tennis shoes, gown, face down with boobs in slots and giant headset), the cancer is Stage 2 because of the size. He says it is 3cm, not 1.6cm, as the ultrasound indicated. Double. Normally, we Southern Californians consider bigger to be better in the bosom. Not today. The MRI also revealed two tiny "satellites" near the primary alien lump.

The BSGI, a newer "97% accurate test" is scheduled for tomorrow. This too, may show if there are additional undetected lumps. Also, we looked at my prior mammograms and although you cannot see Planet Cancer on the September 2009 film, the oncologist thinks it was there, lurking behind dense tissue. How reassuring.

The appointment with the surgeon, Dr. K, is Wednesday at 2:45 p.m. and we will be scheduling my lumpectomy at that time. Surgery: in two to three weeks. Radiation: four weeks after surgery. Simple arithmetic reveals that to be a grand total of seven weeks. Almost springtime.

Monday, January 18th: Later that day: the power of yoga

To everyone who has reached out to me: I am humbled and grateful. Keep it coming!

It is amazing what both Pilates and Yoga do for me. I incessantly preach it to all my students, yet it is true. An hour in the Pilates studio, simply tuning in to breath and movement helped clear my mind. And, relaxed my racing heart. An hour of yoga with Todd (yes, Todd!!) was awesome. I've never actually held hands in Savasana: I highly recommend it.

I'm scared. But, I feel stronger and I will handle this. When I figure out just why I have to handle another tough hurdle, I will let you know. All this experience with death and disease has to serve me somehow, right?

Next week is the ambassador photo shoot for lululemon. I'm really excited, not just to have my big head up on the wall at the store, but to have a positive focus this week. I'm shifting that focus to eating super healthy, not to fight the cancer, but to feel strong and powerful for my photo. I'm stepping up my yoga and Pilates even more for every reason.

It may seem shallow or silly to some, but memorializing myself looking powerful, beautiful (hair and makeup willing), and strong in the setting by the magical ocean I love so much, feels very symbolic. To all the lululemon family: thanks so much for your blessings and support! To everyone in my life: thanks for this love I couldn't have imagined.

Wednesday, January 20th: Update from yesterday and "meet the surgeon" day

Last night, I was so exhausted that not only could I not finish yoga class, but I also couldn't write afterwards. How am I so busy all of a sudden? The whirlwind of appointments is mind-boggling. I thought my pace was rather frenetic before, but wow!

Today I met with the wonderful nutritionist Christa Orecchio. She is a friend and kindly offered to help tweak my diet to turn my body into a cancer-fighting machine. No sugar. Massive greens. Alkaline foods. Flax oil. Organic everything. My brain is very full! I have a terrible sweet tooth and a bad habit of treating myself with cookies when I am a good girl. Chocolate chip, St. Tropez' raspberry heart cookie, Pims dark chocolate with orange, chocolate-dipped shortbread...I could continue. Cookie moratorium for me during treatment. Apparently, sugar is quite the breeding ground for disease. Hell, talking about it makes me want one. Now.

I zoomed over to Seaside Market to purchase the healthy items she recommended. I've never selected a yam before. Interesting looking specimen. We'll see what it looks like when Chef Todd is done with it. As long as it tastes good, I will eat it.

Super greens juice is not tasty. In fact, it is disgusting. I chugged half of it and almost puked in the kitchen sink. I am sorry people, but algae, broccoli, cucumber and whatever other green item was in there does not a tasty drink make. Yuck. I'd much rather eat my veggies. Last night I dreamed about vegetables. I have consumed more leafy greens in the last week than I have in the last month. I cannot help but feel rather virtuous.

Back to the appointment breakdown: the other one was the BSGI test. It is supposed to be an amazingly specific diagnostic test to see if there are any other alien invaders in either breast. Basically, you sit in a chair with one boob on a shelf, while it is photographed from 3 angles, for 7 minutes each. Oh yes, the BSGI started with another dye injection which allowed the camera to reveal a black marble, i.e. the tumor.

The poor technician! She was wonderful, like everyone at Scripps has been, but I guess I talk through those tests in order to not think about them. That woman knows about my childhood living in Africa, my teaching stint for Princeton Review LSAT course, that my sister broke her leg and why she is living in Israel, where Corsica is and why it is a French colony instead of Italian despite Petretti sounding Italian, that my boyfriend is amazing and very different than my past relationships.

Oh yeah, and she also got to arrange my boobs on a shelf several times. Maybe she should have bought me cocktails and dinner? Or, vice versa?

Each appointment must be balanced with an equal or greater beauty treatment. Balance, people, balance! My beauty treat after today's appointment-SPOILER ALERT FOR THOSE WHO THINK MY HAIR GROWS OUT OF MY HEAD THIS WAY-was getting my highlights touched up. Nothing like a little sunshine on the roots to brighten an outlook.

Next, we meet the surgeon and learn, I hope, when she extricates the marble. I am anxious for it to exit stage right. Again, I am super-committed to eating like a champion and creating an invincible immune system, but I want the interloper removed. Period.

Wednesday, January 20th: Not a Lumpectomy!

Apparently, the procedure is called a Partial Mastectomy, not a lumpectomy. I've been corrected by the surgeon, the Nurse Practitioner, the receptionist, and some random person that I'm not even sure works at the hospital. Lumpectomy is not a proper term. It sure sounds better to me. The "M" word scares me.

Today, I was terrified. Whereas part of me felt sure that I'd discovered this early, the other part of me was convinced that I wouldn't escape without them lopping off my boob. My poker face must have failed me again because I was once again offered Xanax. Who knew a cancer diagnosis triggered such an outpouring of various drugs?

To compound the stress further, the nurse called at 2:30 to inform me that the surgeon was running an hour late for my 2:45pm appointment. Seriously? Tick tock. She ended up being almost 2 hours late, necessitating me canceling my 5pm Pilates clients at the last minute. By the time we left Scripps, it was hailing. Yes, there was golf ball sized hail in San Diego. Symbolic much?

I am happy to report that Dr. K not only recommended the lumpectomy (you know what I mean!) and radiation, but also anticipated good results. She showed Todd and me the BSGI and MRI results on her computer screen, which revealed the alien lump lurking inside me. We also saw the 2mm satellite intruder, orbiting nearby. The tests failed to reveal anything else, including the lymph nodes. The tumor is larger than originally diagnosed: 2.5cm. Yet another case of bigger not being better!

Surgery will take place in the next two weeks. Next week, Todd and I escape to Mammoth. I crave a change of scenery. I also desire a smidgen of control, at least in choosing the surgery date!

I finished my evening with lovely, dear friends, without whom I wouldn't be able to keep up my energy and attitude. Yes, I had a glass of wine. If it kills me before surgery, so be it.

Friday, January 22nd: Begone Ye Evil Toxins...

I've had eight appointments in two weeks, not including my beauty treatments to counteract the stress. I've modeled a staggering assortment of gowns, some open in front, some open in back, none in the least flattering. There were also a few capes, resembling mid-arm length ponchos. Again, not my best look. Or anyone's for that matter. My appointment and gown on Thursday were a little different for me: I felt the need to shed poison so I got a colonic. This robe opened in the back for a refreshing change of scenery.

Since my diagnosis, I've had a nagging feeling that I've been poisoned slowly over the years, that toxins have been infiltrating my body. Years of birth control pills, that last keg party at University of Virginia, an occasional In-n-Out burger, non-organic vegetables, Reese's peanut butter cups, who knows?

You could drive yourself insane racking your brain for anything you may have done to create cancer. The bottom line is that I've taken darned good care of myself and this isn't my fault. I refuse to accept responsibility that something I've done in this life caused this cancer.

Neala, my magical facialist, had an excellent observation: perhaps the lump is years of stress: three sibling deaths, my mother leaving when I was 14 years old, my sister's breast cancer, six figure law school loans, divorce, drama, six career changes(okay 10), car accident and resultant neck surgery... the list goes on. My life has been wonderful the last few years with a great relationship and finding my true path career-wise; I believed I had finally reached the easy half. One more bump? But, I digress.

Back to the colonic. I promise not to divulge too much detail. In the past, I've never been drawn to have a colonic but the current toxicity created an almost manic urge to purge. While all the veggies I've consumed the last few weeks have helped, I want more! The lump still lurks within yet I can seize some control. Despite my fear, Lacey at Living Waters in Carlsbad immediately alleviated my fears and I felt safe. She shared her extensive knowledge of the digestive system with me and it made perfect sense. While I did not love the procedure, I love how I felt afterwards. A tune-up.

I decided that while I go through radiation treatment, I'll partake of this procedure weekly. Thus, my liver and gall bladder can excrete the poison as fast as I am filled with it. Whether it actually achieves that result or not, it feels like it is and that is half the battle, right? Silver lining: my stomach feels really flat. Is it bad to enjoy that?

The week's flurry of tests and appointments culminated in Todd surprising me with a romantic dinner at Arterra in Del Mar. After ordering a salad to start and sea bass with more veggies: such a good girl.

Today should be the day that we set the surgery date. I will feel more in control once we do.

Saturday, January 23rd: Ebb and Flow
Ebb and flow. Shadow and light. Good and evil. Dichotomies. Today is definitely ebb. I guess it is all part of a natural cycle, right?

Yesterday, I hit the wall. Not literally, but the impact of body slamming into concrete wall felt real and solid. The adrenaline and manic pace of the last few weeks extracted its toll. When I arrived home, I realized that I hadn't just sat down and relaxed all week. Back to back appointments, information overload, green food obsession and stress plain and simple do not make for a balanced Claire.

Relaxing at home last night helped. Todd and I watched the Haiti telethon and that put things in perspective. I cannot get my head around the reality of the damage in that beaten down country. Why do a vibrant people like the Haitians have to endure that punishment? It is inspiring to see the world helping, to see the optimism in the face of such tragedy.

Back to my own little world. I started this blogging journey and want to finish it, even if it does sometimes seem selfish. Surgery is February 5th. It is outpatient; they say I should be back to yoga and Pilates February 6th.Methinks they don't know the kind of yoga we practice at Sculpt Fusion and Frogs!!But, I'll have the weekend to recover and then plow into February. Then, they give me a four-week reprieve prior to beginning daily radiation treatment for seven weeks. Ugh.

Right now, I am toast. Where will I find the energy for treatment? I was a hot mess in the grocery store with the pressure to find the organic zucchini. Like one regular zucchini will make or break me. All I want right now is a brownie.

My highlight today was teaching the complimentary yoga class at lululemon in Carlsbad. It was my inaugural class as yoga ambassador and it was fantastic. Several of my regular students, friends and the wonderful lululemon family attended to show support and it nourished me.

Thank you, thank you, and thank you for all the love.
Now, I need my own yoga. I'm heading to yoga at 4p.m.in an effort to settle the roiling angst. It is a visceral feeling in my belly at the moment: maybe reality is dawning? Lord knows Denial has been my middle name before. Here's to the upward trend again...

Sunday, January 24th: The Wheatgrass Conspiracy

Re-reading yesterday's entry helps me appreciate how much better I feel today. Yoga helped. Yoga's magic encouraged release of the stored toxins, the stored emotions and the stored trauma from my system.

I admit that I cried in Dandasana, staring down at my cleavage. It was so pretty. I'm realizing that I'm very attached to the girls. They are a part of my identity, my femininity, my body image; one of the few physical traits I share with my sister and mom. Is that shallow? I believe it is deeper than that.

When I had my artificial cervical-disc replacement surgery about fifteen months ago, I was struck by how threatened I felt that the surgeon would be slicing into the front of my throat. Can you say invasive? It feels the exact same way knowing that they'll be wielding the scalpel on my right breast. For some reason, if it were my leg or a less visible body part, it wouldn't be so identity-shaking.

I enjoyed a beautiful morning. The sun is shining again in San Diego and all feels right with the world. The storming and hailing last week contributed to my angst. I'm such a weather wimp, which is probably why I transplanted from Virginia after college. Part of my relocation deal was sunny, at least in the 60s and 70s. All the time. If there is rain, I should be able to stay inside, under a blanket on the couch.

My dear friend Nikke met me at Swamis, a dramatically beautiful beach in Encinitas and we enjoyed a long walk along the pristine coastline. A huge swell is in town due to all the storms and the waves crashed onto the shore. In addition to the seagulls and those little birds with long skinny legs (anyone an ornithologist?), a majestic pelican stood at the edge of the surf: a beautiful, wise old guru. I've never seen one sit there on the beach like a king amongst his subjects. Pelicans are the symbol of forgiveness. Interesting.

After the rejuvenating beach walk, we hit Swamis Café for a yummy, healthy brunch. Christa, my awesome nutritionist, recommended that I take shots of wheat grass at any opportunity. Generally, I've interpreted that to mean if I don't see a billboard posted saying DRINK WHEATGRASS NOW! I can avoid it.

Well, much to my chagrin, Swamis Café had a giant wheat grass sign. Right there on the counter where you order. In plain sight. I couldn't avert my gaze fast enough. Darn it! Nikke took one for the team and we both got a shot. In a word: repulsive. Chills shot from the top of my scalp, down my spine, to the tips of my toes. I cringe just remembering it.

I mean, they have a patch of grass sitting on the counter and they cut it in front of you. I felt like a spoiled rabbit. Ordering my lunch at the counter.

Tuesday, January 26th: Feeling like a "bourrique"

What is a bourrique, you ask? It is a Corsican donkey, famed for its exceptional stubbornness. My grand-père is Corsican and my dad emigrated from France when he was 25.

Quick history lesson: Corsica is a small island in the Mediterranean, the birthplace of Napoleon Bonaparte. Did I mention that not just the bourriques from Corsica are stubborn? The French and Italians fought over ownership for centuries and the French won. Or, so they believe. Corsica is one of the most beautiful places on earth and I was lucky enough to spend several summers of my childhood at my grand-père's flat in L'Ille-Rousse, a magical coastal town.

I digress. Back to why I am fulfilling my father's favorite nickname for me: bourrique(boor-EEK).Currently, I'm feeling very stubborn, resistant, annoyed and rebellious. I'm simply tired of this. Usually, I attack things head-on, knowing very well that I am right and nobody can change my mind. I'm probably quite annoying to be around at times. Thank god my charm and wit balance it out. Ha. Over the last few weeks, I've been determined to find all the best medical advice, holistic advice, survivor advice, diet advice, etc. Now, my brain is overflowing.

When I'm teaching, I'm blessedly released from these obsessive thoughts zooming around my brain. Unfortunately, I teach only a few hours a day. So, the rest of the time I am obsessing about what to eat, what treatment to try, and what book to read next; you get the picture. Not a recipe for calmness and equanimity. I must admit I am enjoying all the veggies, but I am craving a brownie and I must have it or risk going completely batty. Don't try to talk me out of it: I'll butt you with my tough donkey head.

I'm wondering how this disease will affect all my relationships. Everyone has been amazing. My boyfriend is handling this like a champ. He's been taking me to appointments, holding me when I cry, embarking on the organic vegetable adventure with me, trying new recipes, cooking for us, listening to my outbursts and watching me charge through a schedule that cannot be considered sane. I don't want these next few months to be focused solely on my health. Or, our diet. I don't want him to have to shoulder this entire burden. I don't want to be a burden.

My best friend Megan keeps making me cry. We've known each other since we were 14, attended University of Virginia together, and even moved to California together. She knows me better than just about anyone. And, amazingly, still loves me. We have so many funny memories. Her support is rock solid.

The tears seem to be flowing fast and furious: a fellow yoga teacher at Sculpt Fusion Yoga also made me cry today. Her daughter, who has never met me, drew me a picture, complete with chakra colors and her favorite inspirational quotes. She is 13.She also made me a beautiful necklace with a butterfly and a heart.

Again, I am humbled. Family, friends, co-workers, and strangers: so many have reached out to me and all that love and support is fantastic.

Wednesday, January 27th: Adventures of the Masked Yogi at Pre-op

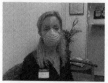

I believed that the hideous gowns and the never-ending boob groping by every employee of Scripps were humiliating enough. But, oh no, was I mistaken.

As you can see by my latest photo, I am not the shallow, vain, boob-obsessed narcissist I may appear to be from my other photo postings. I tried to photo shop my head onto a bikini body shot but alas, I lack the requisite technical skill.

When my friend Joanna and I entered the hospital for the first of three pre-op appointments, we were required to check in with the guardian at the gate. Because I sniffled while we were issued Visitor Badges, said guardian issued me the lovely blue mask I am modeling in my photo. Really? I had to wear it through the hospital to make sure I didn't infect anyone. Very insulting.

Question: why aren't there any air-holes in the mask? I couldn't breathe???!!!

We couldn't stop laughing and I was dying to rip it off but there are cameras everywhere. What if I was kicked out and the surgery delayed? Too risky. After taking this photo opportunity, I stuffed it into my purse. I concocted a good story if we were stopped: the nurse had me remove it to talk and I forgot it in her office...but we exited the hospital through a different door, just to ensure that I didn't have to compromise my integrity!

The gist of today's appointment was to remind me that surgery is scheduled for 12p.m. on Friday, February 5th. Apparently, I will be injected with a painful, radioactive isotope so that when they extract the sentinel lymph node they can see if the cancer has spread. If the cancer has indeed spread, they will remove 10-15 lymph nodes and I will have to wear a drain under my arm for 7-10 days. Is this a joke? How am I to teach hot yoga with a drain under my arm? Sleep? I know they are required to inform me about all the possibilities but this sounds positively medieval.

Joanna played secretary, taking notes as the Nurse Practitioner relayed the details. Thank goodness because these days I have about a 25% retention rate. Kind of like the teacher in the Charlie Brown cartoons. All I seem to recall is "REEEEALLLLYYY PAINFUL INJECTION

INTO YOUR RIGHT BREAST, TAKE XANAX!!! And you "CANNOT EAT OR DRINK 8 HOURS PRIOR TO NOON."How am I not going to eat? I am a monster without my breakfast and every-three-hour feedings. I can only imagine Friday High-Noon: starving, spaced out on Xanax and waiting for surgery. If anyone knows the expedited route to Sainthood, please sign Todd up, as he'll be the one dealing with the hungry beast pre-surgery.

Today marks the fifth recommendation by a hospital employee to take Xanax. And, I am going to follow this advice the day of surgery. Hell, I'm wondering if I should start now?

On a positive note: no more appointments until the actual surgery next week. And, I received the most amazing care package from Colleen Sudduth, a girl I've known since 2nd grade. I cried as I opened it and all the wonderful "moon goddess" goodies, aromatherapy salts, lotions, salves and something called Ass Kisser. Nice.

Friday, January 29th: Jimbo's Juicer Broken...really!

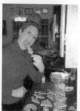

This photo is from Christmas 2009 with Todd's parents. And, yes, I did eat all of those cookies plus a few dozen more! The frosting was green; does that count toward my daily quota of all things green? Or, did all that sugar kick-start my tumor?

Todd and I arrived up in Mammoth Mountain last night. I'm now ensconced under a blanket on the overstuffed

24

couch, with a view of nothing but pristine white snow. What is that phrase? Something bout wherever you go, there you are. Or, you can't run away from your issues? Change of scenery certainly helps, but I have to admit I'm anxious about surgery.

I digress. Imagine that. So, yesterday morning, I'd taught my two back-to-back yoga classes and really needed some nutrition fast. After my healthy bar and some fruit, I wanted an energy boost. Christa, my nutritional advisor had mentioned to go get wheat grass-see my earlier post on my feelings regarding wheat grass-and had mentioned an "uber-energy" drink.

So, I, Claire Petretti, of my own free will, drove to Jimbo's to order the "Emerald Bliss." She did neglect to tell me there was kale involved, but once at the counter I figured I'd just go for it since there were so many other good veggies and apple juice to camouflage the kale. I sauntered up and ordered. With two ounces of wheat grass added no less! Again, I felt rather virtuous because what I really wanted was the package of Deviled Eggs. Fast-forward 10 minutes to the attendant informing me that the juicer was broken and should be repaired in 10 more minutes. Denied! No Emerald Bliss for me!

Well, some may assume that I may have gone for the Deviled Eggs or the tasty looking cranberry muffin that beckoned. Nope. I actually purchased the Evolution Essential Greens. Yes, the same vegetable juice combination that gave me dry heaves just one short week ago. I guzzled the entire bottle in the car, without a gag or a gasp. I did, however, have a greenish ring around my mouth. Kind of like when you drink yummy chocolate milk. Just without the yumminess.

That's all from the mountain. One week from today will provide answers. Until I wake up from the surgery Friday afternoon and know that I don't have a drain under my arm that signals that the cancer has spread, I won't be able to truly relax.

Saturday, January 30th: Kale, kale, everywhere

Okay, there is a kale conspiracy. Yes, just like the bloody wheatgrass. My mother used to boil kale and douse it with vinegar. Needless to say, eating that is an experience that stays with you forever. Kale is also an excellent food for iguanas: they thrive on it. To me, kale is intended as lunch for iguanas. I am not an iguana. Vitamins be damned.

After lazing about all day yesterday, except for 90 minutes of yummy yoga while Todd snowboarded, we descended into the village and enjoyed an excellent dinner.

I chose the ono for dinner, but a huge dilemma ensued. According to the menu, the ono was served on a bed of kale. I asked our throwback to Fast Times at Ridgemont High-looking waiter if the chef would substitute the broccolini for the kale. Denied!

Apparently, the chef at Petra's is an artiste and refuses to make substitutions that might mar the integrity of his creations. Broccolini: NO. Broccolini was served only with the New York Steak. No broccolini for you! Soup Nazi anyone? With a little finagling, I managed to procure spinach. HA!! I swear, I have never seen, heard or smelled so much kale in my life.

Today, I feel good. I've finally relaxed a bit and feel like I am on vacation. Todd and I started the morning with some yoga. For the first time in the history of visiting a ski resort town, I am not going to ski or snowboard. Now, for those of you who have witnessed me skiing or snowboarding: stop laughing! Although my descent may not win me any medals, I have fun. For some reason, I just don't have the strength to attempt it.

Instead, we are going sledding! You can't go to the snow without careening down the mountain and laughing like a maniac. That is the plan! Sledding will be followed by a cozy dinner at the condo. R&R before the surgery.

Sunday, January 31st: Misadventures in the Mystic Booth

I am officially losing my marbles (except that damn one that I'd like to lose).The last one hit the floor folks. My episode du jour confirmed it. Good news: the hilarity saved me from a complete meltdown. What a trade-off. Quid pro quo (I do remember some legalese) I laughed so hard at myself that it provided me a short respite from the darkness permeating my being.

After a relaxing weekend in the winter wonderland that is Mammoth, I had one important task tonight: to get a tan. A mystic tan. My long-awaited ambassador photo shoot for lululemon is Tuesday morning and I want to look my best. I'm not sure why this photo is so symbolic for me but it is. Strength, power, beauty.

One negative aspect to the vacation weekend was all the uninterrupted time to think. And, the path my mind traveled was a morbid, morose spiral. I am officially freaking out. I don't know if it is finally dawning on me that I have CANCER and suddenly I have no clue how I can maintain my sanity until surgery Friday. Until I surface from anesthesia, I will not know if the cancer has spread. Nothing but the biopsy of the sentinel lymph node can confirm whether this evil alien has spread its seed. No pressure. No pressure at all.

Unable to battle the Xanax pushers any longer, I finally succumbed, taking Xanax to sleep. Bizarre, unpleasant dreams filled my restless slumber. No more. I will take a Valium on Friday pre-surgery but that is it. Maybe the Xanax has an after-effect of lowering my IQ because I am not the sharpest tool in the shed at the moment.

Okay, enough morbidity. Here's the funny story.

Back in the day, I was the mystic tan master. I've been using that Porta-potty-looking booth that sprays you and leaves you a lovely golden tan for eons. A tan without getting any sun damage! Fabulous! Over the years, I learned all the little tricks to avoid getting streaked hands, orange feet and all the other potential side-effects that mar your glow if you fail to be vigilant with your exfoliation, your barrier cream, your hand position... I could go on forever. No mistakes here.

Granted, I haven't gotten a mystic tan in a while. All the wheatgrass consumption and groping by hospital employees leaves little time for worrying about a golden glow. Regardless, the blunder I made tonight was a first.

I was distracted. I brought a bikini bottom but, it never made it out of my purse.

Oblivious to that little snafu, I was in the booth, shower cap in place, ready to get golden. I pushed the Start button.

Cold spray shot out from the nozzles, dousing me from head to toe. I looked down and screamed.

My Bra. Was. On. My Boobs. Not only had I forgotten to put on my bikini bottoms, but I'd also forgotten to take off my bra.

I ripped the offending garment off and tossed it on the floor of the booth. Of course, I'd asked for the bronzing version of the tan and my bra turned a lovely shade of brown. Oops... I hope I caught it in time or I'll have some funny strap marks in my photographs.
Yes, that was the last marble.

Chapter 2: February

Tuesday, February 2nd: 2 down, 3 to go

All I remember about Monday was gagging down the Emerald Bliss from Jimbo's. Garnished with two shots of wheat grass. The Emerald Bliss should be renamed Bitter Bile. I was proud of myself for my persistence after the broken juicer incident last week. It took me 45 minutes to consume half of the 16 ounces. Disgusting. I'd rather graze on grass on the side of the highway. It would probably be more pleasant. Thank goodness Monday is over.

This morning was fabulous: my long-awaited photo shoot for my lululemon ambassador photo that will hang in the Carlsbad store right above the yoga pants.

Becoming an ambassador has been a goal of mine for the last few years. Ever since my dear friend Angie Stewart-Goka became an ambassador for lululemon in Beverly Hills, I was intrigued by the program. Lululemon, for those of you who aren't up on your popular yoga apparel, is an amazing yoga and fitness apparel company built on principles of community.

Health, wellness, living in the present moment, making the most of each second of the day: it resonates! As an ambassador, I represent lululemon in the community and am also recognized by them as a Yoga and Pilates professional that embodies their values.

Ambassadors have a large photo on the wall of the store and I love that! Once a Leo, always a Leo. But, it became significantly more meaningful to me after my diagnosis.

Memorializing Claire pre-surgery is powerful. We shot at the beach in South Carlsbad. Sunrise was amazing, although I was freezing my tail off!!Sitting on ice plant and balancing on the cliff edge over the ocean makes a pretty picture but it was cold. Oh, the price we pay. I loved having the lululemon ladies Laura, Sherry and Meredith there to ensure all went smoothly and Tai the photographer was great.

Teaching went well today and I had time for a nap. Jake and Oreo were thrilled that I'd seen the light and finally understood that afternoons are best spent snuggling and sleeping. I love my kitties: simple, pure affection.

Day 2 of this week down, 3 to go. I've got Wednesday and Thursday tightly scheduled to minimize brooding.

Wednesday, February 3rd: Day One Too Many

If I didn't have my teaching, I would be completely insane. My yoga and Pilates students are absolutely amazing and remind me every day why I left corporate America. Sharing positive energy and knowing that I am helping them as much as they are helping me is incredibly powerful. Everyone at Sculpt Fusion Yoga has been so warm and caring, giving me an incredible amount of support and love. Thank you, thank you, and thank you.

I cannot fathom what this experience would have been like if I still sold legal and business software or God forbid, still practiced law. Can you imagine? "Claire, I know you are having surgery Friday so, can you come in Sunday to make up your billable hours please?"

I feel like I'm biding my time. Only one doctor's appointment: Surgery. Day after tomorrow. Tick tock. Tick tock. TGIF, in the sense that I'll know if the cancer has spread on Friday afternoon.

I've been staying really busy and the condo would definitely pass the white glove test. I'm talking mopped floors, washed rugs, sparkling refrigerator drawers. The flurry of activity helped me not think. Key to sanity: chittavrittinirodhah. Sanskrit for stilling the fluctuations of the mind.

I feel strong, supported, loved and optimistic. I'm still pissed off that I have this disease. Furious. Cancer, Cancer, Cancer. What the hell? I did actually have someone say to me that I was lucky that it was "just breast cancer."

Are you kidding me? Just because now one in eight women has breast cancer, up from one in 20 only 30 years ago, doesn't make it less of a tragic disease. Yes, it is treatable; yes, the survival rates are high but people die from it every day.

And it's painful to go through no matter the outcome. A yoga student gave me an article called "The Unbearable Lightness of Breast Cancer" written by a survivor who was appalled at how every woman stricken with the disease was expected to put on a happy face, don pink, and make the best of it. She was outraged at the lack of anger. Hear, hear!

I am the type of person who makes things work. No matter what. I've been labeled a Survivor and never liked the term. Life isn't something to be survived, it should be savored. Unfortunately, the savoring portion has been lacking in 2010. I will deal with it. I'll be strong. But, I don't have to like it and I'm not going to pretend that it is "just breast cancer." I feel like I should add "So there!"

It is time to curl up in the freshly laundered sheets with Jake and Oreo and attempt to read. It is frustrating: my favorite pastime of reading has been marred by my shortened attention span.

Thursday, February 4th: Surgery Eve: Time to put on the Granny Panties

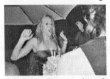

This photo is from my 40th birthday party in Beverly Hills. What a fun night! I remember this moment clearly. I remember exactly what I wished for when I blew out my candles.

I wished for true love, I wished to find purpose and direction in my career, I wished to get rid of drama in my life, I really wished the cake to be chocolate inside, I wished to keep all the beautiful friends and family in my life who have always been there for me. And, every single wish was granted. Every single wish. But, I forgot to make a wish for my health...Tonight; I will blow out a candle wishing for health, in addition to maintaining the rest of my wonderful, blessed rollercoaster of a life.

You've heard the phrase in a crisis situation: "It is time to put on your Big Girl Panties."Today even the big girl panties won't suffice: time for the Granny Panties. And the matching bra.

Surgery Eve doesn't have quite the same impact as Christmas Eve or even Birthday Eve, my personal favorite. Yet, a similar anticipation exists. The same inability to relax, the same fear of not sleeping, the same wonder of what will be unwrapped is tangible. Definitely an Ambien-night. Watch me end up addicted to Ambien. Sleep is vital at this point by whatever means.

I must confess that my immediate concern is that I cannot eat after midnight and I don't check in for surgery until 12pm.Really??!! I'm going to starve. If I don't get fed every two to three hours, the results are ugly. I'd even take a kale shake!

Tonight, Todd is treating us to a delicious dinner at my favorite Italian restaurant. Here is the mastermind plan: gorge myself with pasta, bread and whatever isn't nailed down to the table, bring home leftovers and devour a second feeding right before midnight. I am shrinking and not in a pretty way. I swear, the only thing that makes me lose weight is a break-up or cancer. All the nervous energy and all the veggies... is that the silver lining?

So, I am prepared for tomorrow:

Health Care Directive: Check.
- List of phone numbers for Todd to call after surgery: Check.
- My surgery outfit (just like you lay out your outfit on Christmas Eve for the big night). - Maybe I will be able to convince myself that tomorrow is Christmas: Check.
- Fuzzy purple "slipper-socks," courtesy of my friend Anaise: Check.
- Rolling Stones vintage zip-front sweatshirt: Check.
- My favorite fancy white sweat pants: Check. And...
- The nurse directed me to bring a sports bra that closes in front for my après-surgery ensemble. I could only find one that cost $50 and it was atrocious. I'm talking hideous. I am sorry, but I am not spending $50 on something that an 85 year old grandmother would find frumpy!!So, I went to Target and got a $10 regular front close bra. It should work, right? They can stuff me and whatever is left of my bosom right into it. And seal me in with Mick Jagger's lips.

I received a highly entertaining care package today. Lots of healing positive items, including a Dr. Seuss book and my favorite: a small "beck and call" bell so I don't have to bellow for bon-bons. How have I made it this far in life without that bell?? Thank you, Anaise. It is fabulous!! Todd may beg to differ by the end of the weekend...

I feel grateful. Very spoiled, pampered and loved. The outpouring of support is keeping me buoyant despite the situation. And, I love hearing from some old friends that I haven't spoken to in a years. Amazing how friendship lasts and memories never fade. An old sorority sister reminded me that Meg and I used to have a preference for jugs of Peach Riunite wine in college. How our tastes have evolved!!

Time to sign off and prepare for a romantic date with the love of my life. I'm not sure if I will write pre-surgery tomorrow or not. Thanks for listening and allowing me this forum.

Friday, February 5th: Definitely not Christmas or my Birthday

I just popped some painkillers, drained the disgusting grenade-looking drain under my arm and am sitting here, devastated. Oreo is on my lap. Not up to talking quite yet but figured I'd write.

I did not anticipate waking up with a drain under my arm and everything that the stupid, disgusting thing signifies. The cancer spread to the lymph nodes and that means in all probability chemotherapy and radiation. Is this numbness shock?

When I woke up from anesthesia, I was in excruciating pain. It was as if someone speared an ice pick through my breast. Grading the pain scale was simple: 10 out of 10.

Next, I realized that there was a drain and in that instant my world shattered.

Usually, percentages are my friend. Not today. Statistically, there was a 10 percent chance that the cancer had spread to the lymph nodes. For once, being in the top 10 percent stinks. In the past, I've strived to excel, never doing anything halfway. Top percentile in IQ, top percentile in body fat percentage, top spelling bee in elementary school. Hell, even top percentile for some of my old sales jobs, although that was only luck.

What I wouldn't do to be in the middle of the bell curve right now.

I've always lived life on a big scale. No halfway. Again, I really wish that wasn't the case right now. Couldn't I have been part of the 80% with a benign lump? Among the 90% that hadn't spread?

Yes, I am "Why me-ing" right now. I'm sure I'll move on, but it is all I feel right now.

Let's see: silver lining. Digging deep here: Todd did stop and get us Mish-Mosh soup from Milton's and it was yummy and perfect. Oreo is still on my lap and his purring is making me happy. The forecast calls for rain all weekend and for once, I am glad. It fits.

I am sure that I will pull myself up and beat the crap out of this. But, I really wish that I just didn't have to fight.

Saturday, February 6th: Not much to report...

The "Why me?" trend continues.

Because the drain continues to leak, I'm sporting Outfit #3 of the day. Last night, I soaked through the ace bandage the doctor wrapped me in so, I sent Todd out to get the previously recommended hideous sports bra.

Let's try to find some positive: thanks for all the wonderful messages, calls and emails. You are amazing. Thanks Steve and Carol for the beautiful flowers, thanks Kim for more beautiful flowers, thanks Jessie for the Emerald Bliss sans wheatgrass (much better!) and chocolate covered strawberries, thanks Zoe for your love, empathy, support and having a daughter that is a girl scout. Thanks Anni for setting me up with your healer in LA. Most of all, thanks to Todd for playing nursemaid to a miserable patient.

Please keep calling and writing. It lifts me up.

My sister and dad are coming to visit on the 23rd and I am so grateful for the opportunity to see them. I hope my brother can come too.

Where is the fast-forward button? I want to know my exact treatment protocol, my completion date, how, when, what, why. God give me the strength to endure this.

Sunday, February 7th: Drain, drain, go away

Drain, drain, go away, never come back any day.

Poetry has never been my forte. Neither has patience. Seriously, this drain is unquestionably the worst part of this experience thus far. Far worse than the radioactive isotope-thingy they shot into my boob pre-surgery. The injections were painful but this drain is disgusting. Worse than looking at the bandage and imagining what lay beneath. Have I made my point?

Earlier today, little black dots floated before my eyes when we were going for Sports Bra #4. I almost collapsed when I made the mistake of actually looking at where the drain was emerging out of my underarm. Not a good idea.

The drain wasn't draining properly and I've been soaking through all these clothes, towels, and sheets. I called the hospital today and the nurse on call asked me if I'd been "stripping the drain"…um, no. No idea what that means. Long story short: you are supposed to pull on the drain 3 or 4 times without pulling it out of the skin completely. Sure, that is intuitive. How would I know to do that?

Then, I'm supposed to stay compressed in the hideous sports bra to help the healing process, the internal stitches, etc. But, the stupid thing was so tight that I think it blocked the drainage tube. Another lululemon sports bra is toast. This is becoming expensive. Because I couldn't breathe in the hideous zippered contraption, I decided to step into a slightly oversized lululemon bra and pull it up. Success! My achievement for the day.

I had a nightmare. Drugs will do that to you. I dreamt that they called me from lululemon and told me that they were putting my ambassadorship on hold because of all the upcoming treatment. I was devastated. After all I went through in the mystic tan booth.

My life is on hold. I can't teach until this drain is removed. I can't leave the house until the drain is removed. Once the drain is gone, who knows what the future holds?

How can I not go insane? Taking it day by day is impossible when I look down at this drain, impossible as I cannot indulge in my former favorite escape of reading because I now have the attention span of a gnat, impossible because I don't know what they are going to tell me on Tuesday regarding recommended treatment protocols.

I'm not ready to "begin the fight" right now. I don't feel like activating my inner warrior to get fired up for battle. I'm exhausted. I've been fighting my entire life and I really want to just "be" for the second half.

And, by just "being", I mean publishing a novel, publishing more health and wellness articles and a book, succeeding on ExerciseTV, helping others through my teaching, living on a LARGE scale. I've finally found my calling after my forays through law, sales, and charity work. Damn it! I don't have time to deal with this disease. I have too much to do. I've finally found my man. I'm just getting started and this whole cancer bullshit is very inconvenient.

When I first got the diagnosis, I was very pragmatic: I will get the lump removed, get my radiation, which will be annoying and time-consuming, but, I will be done in time to go to Australia with Todd in May. Boom, boom, boom. Get it done. This evil drain is sucking away my plans.

A wise woman suggested that I sit back for the ride and allow others to fight for me. It sounds good. I am humbled by all the offers of help from those close to me and those who really aren't that close to me too. I need to learn to receive. How?

Monday, February 8th: Support makes all the difference

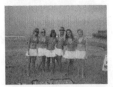

and not just in the sports bras! RIP to the bra above: this is the one I sliced open and hooked with safety pins prior to breaking down and having Todd fetch me the giant recommended hideous harness.

I woke up this morning feeling much better. Perhaps the fact that the damn drain isn't soaking everything helps a great deal. But, I think that the collective energy I've been receiving massaged me with magical hands overnight and the healing has begun. How did I get to be so lucky and not have to travel this path alone? All of the comments on the blog help me.

In response to Jenny L's blog comment regarding my lack of patience: no, patience is not and never has been my virtue. Most of my friends and other unsuspecting listeners have heard my rants while I am driving (impatiently).Usually something along the lines of, "la la la, I'm going to teach my favorite yoga class right now, feeling really Zen...YOU STUPID G--D---MO--FO--LEARN TO DRIVE!!!!!." Sorry, but these people need to pay attention and learn how to drive. My Corsican blood cannot be denied. No matter how calm and happy I feel, the bad drivers get me every time. Oh well, nobody is perfect, right?

Today, I feel semi-normal and am going to wean off these meds. I'm not sure how I will feel tomorrow when I get the results of the lymph node dissection. I am praying that the evil alien hasn't been able to infiltrate very far past the sentinel node. Perhaps that extra-virtuous shot of wheatgrass I had last week blocked its progress. Perhaps the Emerald Bliss will prevent it too. I'm visualizing all these greens acting like shields, battling the nasty creepy mold-like infiltrators.

I'm going to enjoy today and have Todd walk me around the block now. Some sun and fresh air has to help.

My arm feels very weird. The right shoulder and upper half of my arm feels numb. Is that lymphedema? I hope it dissipates soon.

I hope that when the drain comes out I can teach. Maybe Thursday or Friday? Then again, I don't know what I'll feel like when they give me the recommended treatment protocol. The not knowing and waiting is tough.

Okay, going to try to just focus on the present.

Tuesday, February 9th: How to stuff a watermelon into...

The morning was not an auspicious start to the day. Imagine trying to stuff a watermelon into your nostril.

No, wait. Imagine trying to stuff me, the godforsaken drain that I cannot stop complaining about, and several gauze sponges into an old sports bra with just two arms. First, I tried the "stripping the drain" because I could see blood clots and it was leaking. Gross, gross, gross. In my awkward attempts, I practically yanked the drain out by accident, which resulted in me almost fainting and vomiting simultaneously. Dizzy with pain and frustration, I howled like a wolf a few times, thus scaring the cats, who were watching the entire process quizzically. They prefer when I nap with, feed, or pet them.

42

This hellish endeavor lasted almost forty minutes and by the time I was done, I was angry and close to tears. And, because I'd decided to stop taking the Percocet today, I was in severe pain.

A generous friend offered to not only take me to a healer she knew, but also to drive me to LA to see her. When she picked me up, she had an Emerald Bliss for me. Ugh. It doesn't get tastier people. Trust me. Anyway, I was not a happy girl when she picked me up or when we arrived in Hollywood for the appointment.

It went well, although I didn't have that immediate connection or resonance that you sometimes have with people. The healer told me immediately that I needed to let go of the anger and resentment in order to start healing. That directive may take some work because I remain devastated about waking up with the drain. Defeat emanated from every pore.

After the session, I felt more like myself. Not quite feisty, but somehow lighter and less hopeless. The drain continues to leak and the feeling is returning to my shoulder. Unfortunately, it is shooting electric shockwaves, but nonetheless it isn't numb.

I called twice for the pathology results and was lectured by the nurse. No, the results won't be ready today. No, (you annoying little pest as I told you yesterday!) they probably won't be ready tomorrow. The earliest is Thursday. So, I will call again tomorrow.

All the other results were ready earlier than they expected. I am praying that the cancer did not spread beyond the sentinel node and that all those nodes they removed will be clear. So, only radiation needed. I cannot face the alternative.

I want the drain removed so I can start moving like myself again. So, I can consider moving around and teaching again. It seems very far away at the moment. Recalling balancing on my right arm in side plank last week is a distant dream.

Wednesday, February 10th: Showering can be fun

Incredible what stopping Percocet will do for your psyche. Pain meds do not make me a happy girl. I may be repeating myself. I should probably go back and read my prior entries. Here I am thinking I'm learning something new every day and perhaps I'm just repeating myself. And rambling.

Today was exponentially better than yesterday. And so on. Saturday, that nightmare blur of leaking drains, teary eyes and sheer despair seems far away. I feel more like me. Less like the defeated, sad little shell of Claire. I can't help but talk about myself in the third person because throughout these last weeks, it is as if I've been watching myself in a movie. Even with my vivid imagination, I couldn't have scripted this.

I am ready for the results and ready for the removal of the drain.

In the meanwhile, I've discovered how to shower with the drain without yanking it numerous painful times. You kneel. Or squat. Or for the yogis out there, take malasana. This position prevents the drain from pulling out the opening in your flesh. The possibilities are endless in malasana, like washing your hair, adding conditioner, rinse and repeat. Do not, I repeat, do not attempt to shave your legs.

I do need help. I need someone to shave my right armpit.

Those who know me well know that grooming is very important to me. As is balance. How can I have one hairy armpit with a drain coming out? I'm sorry, a numb, hairy armpit. Not pretty. Not like I am at my sexiest these days: but the armpits need to be cleared. Any volunteers? I am serious.

I continue to receive lovely messages, visitors, gifts and support. I continue to be blown away by it all. The Camp women rock. Everyone rocks!

I must comment that I feel very popular. Sorry if that is dorky, but if we were in high school, I'd win Homecoming Queen, no contest. And, I didn't get that first time around. I am so happy, so blessed, so warm inside at all the love. And, lucky for me, Todd was Quarterback so; he knows how to escort the HQ.

I'm off to start my New Moon puzzle. Maybe I'll put in the Twilight soundtrack while I do it. Or, the New Moon soundtrack. Decisions, decisions.

Thursday, February 11th: Foot massages rock

Today was a good day, despite still having the drain that keeps on draining. For the drain to be removed, I must secrete less than 30ccs of whatever nasty substance is exiting my hairy underarm for 2 consecutive days. I've already had 75ccs today. Thus, we are already out to Sunday at a minimum. Arg!

No teaching Monday. But I cannot teach while the evil drain remains intact.

No test results. Take your time pathology lab, take your time.

No hurry.

Luckily, today was full of wonderful visits and calls. My dear friend Angie drove down from LA with her faithful companion Puffy to bring me lunch and flowers. How cool is that? I am so spoiled. She also walked me. She had Puffy on one arm, me on the other. Well, I exaggerate. I walked without a leash, but still feel like I'm being walked, as opposed to going for a walk. It is beautiful outside, sunny, clear and breezy. It felt good to be outside, if only for a brief stroll.

As Angie exited stage left, Carmel entered, with a beautiful tray of fresh veggies and fruits and her massage tools: two strong hands. Since I still have the godforsaken drain in and we couldn't do a full massage, Carmel gave me the most amazing foot massage.

Reminds me of Pulp Fiction and one of my favorite scenes, no, not "look at the big brain on Brad," but when John Travolta and Samuel L. Jackson debate the art of foot massage. If Carmel had worked her magic on Mia Wallace's feet, I'm sure Marcellus would have had her tossed out of a window too. Amazing. Thank you, thank you!!!

We briefly debated wigs, should that be an issue in the upcoming months (no, no, no).I did decide I want big hair. I'm talking late 1980s, spiral perm. Big, fluffy: Tawny Kitaen in the Whitesnake video. But, that isn't going to be an issue. Just in case.

My day's activities took me out of the house for the first time. Back to Living Waters and Lacy for my après-surgery colonic. I feel like I managed to purge some of that anesthesia, Valium, Percocet and Ambien. Who knew that I would find it so soothing, but it feels very powerful to have some control of ridding my body of poisons.

46

Todd arrived home earlier than expected, which made me very happy. We shared a quiet night before the big Post-op appointment tomorrow. Fingers crossed that we've got results and they are what we want to hear. Clear, clear, clear.

Friday, February 12th: One leap forward, two steps back...Post-op

Okay, I'm trying to be positive because I was wishing, wishing, wishing that the remaining lymph nodes were clear and they are. I am very pleased that it hasn't infiltrated further into my body.

So, one node of ten is positive. My sister had eight positive ones, so that gives me a benchmark. Her treatment was brutal--she is the strongest woman I know and survived, but it hurt every moment to see what she had to endure.

I thought that just one teeny-weeny, itsy-bitsy, little node would mean no chemotherapy, but the doctor extinguished that hope by pointing out that:

1) It is still positive
2) It still metastasized
3) and that even though it didn't get far, she believes chemo will be in order

Epiphany of the day: once a lawyer, always a lawyer. I found myself negotiating with the doctor to avoid chemo. Once again, the scenario felt surreal, as if I were watching myself star in a nightmare. How many ways can Claire reframe the question until she gets the answer she wants? Unfortunately, my persistence failed to pay off with the desired response.

Next week, we meet with the medical oncologist, who is the dictator of the "recipe" for further treatment. My best friend's mom Judy, who is like a second mother to me, has been incredibly helpful and supportive through this process, sharing knowledge from her invaluable background as an oncology nurse. She explained that they make up a unique cocktail/recipe based on a variety of factors, not just the positive lymph node. Great.

In order to avoid going completely batty, I will research alternatives to that dreaded C. I remain reluctant to believe it is the true solution. I know it kills the cancer cells, but so many people I've seen go through it never have the same immune system again. Instead, I can only see the permanent poisoning of my entire system. But, I will attempt to listen to the oncologist with an open mind. I am not ruling it out but I am not committing to it.

Again, let me emphasize that I am grateful that the cancer did not spread farther. But I also need time to process what I call the two steps back. There is no black and white. Shades of gray. And, I hope people can understand and respect my need to acknowledge and process the enormity of this terrible news.

Sometimes, life just sucks. No silver lining. No false cheer. Optimism tempered by pragmatism? Who knows? Perhaps I'll be enlightened by the end of this process. Again, I cannot pretend that I am not devastated by some of today's news.

When they performed my lumpectomy, they took out margins of healthy tissue surrounding the tumor. Apparently, they now have to go back in for a second surgery because they failed to get clear margins on the section of the lump where the "satellite" tumor was. So, they have to open me back up, go in and "shave off" a little more flesh. More anesthesia. More surgery.

Seriously? This will most likely occur in two weeks. Really? All that for one centimeter and a half?

In addition, this godforsaken drain remains attached until at least Tuesday. I cannot teach. I cannot start any physical therapy on the arm that refuses to budge beyond shoulder height. I cannot wear anything that pulls over my head. On a humorous note, the doctor suggested I put the drain in a fanny pack and blouse my top out over it. Granted, she's only seen me in a hospital gown or she would know I don't own anything that would blouse out over said fanny pack. I refuse to buy new clothes to dress the drain. Nor am I buying a fanny pack.

Also, I learned that my underarm will be permanently numb. And, they want me to wear a sleeve whenever I fly because of barometric pressure changes--not sure if that is forever too. Apparently, some nerves are "sacrificed" to take out the lymph nodes. I get to be fitted for said sleeve. I am sure that will be interesting.

So, back to the positive: it only spread to one node. My dear old friend Robert came by and did some healing energy work and I took a lovely peaceful nap with Jake. Todd is home and came to the appointment with me and I feel lucky to have his unwavering support. I received more amazing care packages: I am SPOILED. Love it. I now have a stuffed bunny and an angel bear watching out for me.

The drain remains and the armpit continues to sprout hair...maybe I can grow it long enough to do a comb over if necessary down the road?

Saturday, February 13th: Even the Big Girl Panties don't cover the drain

Okay, I risk redundancy with my obsession with the drain but I cannot hide it, I cannot escape it, I certainly cannot pretend that it isn't there. It is a tangible, daily reminder that something. is. really. wrong.

Please enjoy the photo of said drain, which omits the spot where it comes out of my upper ribcage because that is too repulsive to share. Just follow that long, blood-clotted tube up to a hole about two inches below my hairy armpit. Oh yes, don't forget the gauze bandages taped to my skin to absorb the leaks.

This week will be marked by a Remove the Drain Party. I'm going to ask the doctor to release the drain to take home with me. I'd like a big ritual. A dramatic ritual. Environmentally friendly of course. Stab it, whack it with a bat, chop it, you name it--I am open!! I'm not usually an advocate for violence but I think that this drain needs a beating. Todd suggested stringing it up like a piñata...now we are on the right track!

In this disease with shades of gray, I think killing the drain is a healthy symbol of black and white. I've had to surrender so much, to have faith in a questionable future with uncertain remedies; I'd like to have something concrete. Like obliterating this symbol of doom.

As for the rest of today, it has been lovely. I continue to chafe in my confinement. We did go for a walk at Batiquitos lagoon, however. I love that place. It is a beautiful trail where you can enjoy the kiss of the ocean breeze, watch egrets and ducks while away the day, and be surrounded by trees and pure nature. And, San Diego hit 69 degrees and sunny today. I love living here.

More visitors today: thank you Randi and Lauren! Randi made us the most incredible vegetarian organic chili. It was truly the best chili I've ever had. Todd and I stuffed ourselves. Oink.

Then, Lauren brought me the latest trashy gossip magazine. And an Emerald Bliss. I forgot how those tasted. The evil Jimbo's juice maker wouldn't cut the bitterness with a banana. He is a bad person. But, I'm boosting my immune system. Green, green, green. I feel like with the help of my friends, I am doing all I can to fight this cancer with nutrition. Lots of vegetables, Super Greens, and Girl Scout cookies. Balance, right?

La piece de resistance: Lisa sent me the cat hat that I found and failed to purchase!! Lisa--how did you find it? I love it. I am the cat lady in the cat hat. :) Most people who know me recognize that I am the crazy old cat lady in training. I don't see any issue with letting the rest of the world know. It isn't like I have anything to hide these days.

Sunday, February 14th: Research and Risk/Benefit Rations...getting technical on this cancer

A brilliant artist named Campbell Morin took this upside down photo. Granted, Campbell was missing her two front teeth and still measures her age in one digit but genius knows no age limits! Thanks Angel Bear!

Today is the day I got serious about my research. All those years of learning, using, and selling legal research will finally be useful. My goal is to have as much credible information as possible prior to meeting the oncologist on Friday. I will also definitely set up a second opinion. I'm compiling my list of questions for the doctor. I'd love to find someone who will tell me I don't have to have chemotherapy. Calling once? Calling twice? Please?

A friend gave me *How to Prevent and Treat Cancer with Natural Medicine,* by Dr. Michael Murray. After reading it, I've tabbed the four most immediately pertinent chapters for Todd to review. And, I numbered them in order of priority. With hot pink post-its.

What is excellent about this resource is that it doesn't advise forgoing conventional treatments such as surgery, chemo, radiation and drugs. Rather, it advises how to best use nutrition, diet and natural supplements to boost your immune system, stay strong and complement other treatments. There are numerous studies on greens and antioxidants, among other holistic remedies.

No question exists regarding the paramount importance of nutrition. Surgery helps. Medicine helps. Acupuncture helps. Healing work helps. Yoga helps. Prayer helps. Love helps. The resounding support that I've received definitely helps.

There is no single cure-all.

I fail to be convinced that chemotherapy is The Cure. I am open to hearing the arguments pro and con. What is the individual prognosis for a 43-year-old, very healthy, Stage 2 ER/PR positive cancer with one positive lymph node?

I demand statistics. What are the survival/recurrence rates if I do surgery and radiation only? What are they if I do surgery, radiation and chemotherapy? What about the hormone drugs? What if I do nothing else after the second surgery? What if I sell my car and travel for the next few months instead?

What are the success rates? Ratios? Side effects? What is the risk/benefit ratio?

What are the long-term effects to my immune system? This concerns me greatly. Do I want to live an extra five years but have a cold or infection every month? Or, would I rather live out the rest of my days healthy and strong? How is quality of life considered?

Quality over quantity.

I'm finding that I straddle the natural and conventional theories and want to maximize both. I won't swallow an entire recommendation without questioning it. I won't decide out of fear. I will do this my way. No guarantees exist for any of this.

I cannot suppress my anxiety about work. When do I get to return to teaching? And, how much more time will be sacrificed for treatment? It isn't just that if I don't work I don't get paid. I'm in the process of building my Pilates clientele. This damn cancer is an unwelcome interruption. I want the Drain Out so I can return to yoga and Pilates. I cannot lift my right arm above shoulder height and I'm having some sharp pain in my arm and underarm. The numb one.

How can it be numb and hurt too? Paradox.

Ending on a positive note: Happy Valentine's Day! I got to spend a leisurely day with my Valentine. Watching the sunset over the Pacific with the man I love is such a gift.

Monday, February 15th: Time to let me out...

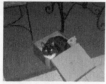

This is Oreo. He loves curling up in little boxes where he can nap leaning against the walls. He will remain there, safe and cozy, all day. While I appreciate his feelings, I do not share them. I feel trapped. I have had one daily supervised outing each day for a walk. Like a pet. Other than that, this drain has chained me indoors.

I'm going batty. I know, I know, I know! The drain is serving an honorable service by removing the fluids and toxins from my body. I get it. I appreciate it. Give it a medal. But, if I have to measure these fluids and record them, if I have to get a stringy blood clot stuck on my finger as I empty said fluids, one more time, I will snap. I've lost count of how many times I've almost passed out or thrown up. Or both. Ten days is a long time. And, it isn't coming out Tuesday so, we are at Wednesday already.

I'm used to running around all day. I teach all over North County. Some might think my usual pace is frenetic, but I thrive on it. I've never been one to sit around the house. Currently, I have the attention span of a turnip. I love to read. You'd think I'd have devoured ten books by now, but I cannot seem to focus. Like a hamster running on its wheel, my brain continues to circle the cancer ride.

Luckily, in addition to my walk, I had two visitors today. My old friend Anne came bearing tons of organic veggies and great conversation. Robert came by for my second pranic healing session. I'm hitting this cancer from every angle possible.

No profound insights today. Just biding time and trying to take it one day at a time.

Wednesday, February 17th: Bye-Bye Drain

It is Wednesday and the drain continues to hang around. This morning, I was thrilled to wake up and glance down at the drain and see it was almost empty. I bounded downstairs to measure my lymphatic fluid output. Only 5cc! Earlier on in this process, I'd wake up with 30ccs and not be quite so eager to measure it because it meant further imprisonment. Today will be twelve days. The drain has been the most challenging part of this process thus far.

To be honest, since I set up the appointment to have the drain removed today, I've been scared that it would start flowing again and I would have to keep it longer. I'm not used to operating with so much fear in my life. I'm generally pretty fearless and I am not comfortable in the role of wimp. So, I have been a crabby little brat. You know when you hear yourself and think, "Shut Up!" but you keep ranting anyway? Can you say Harpy? Thank goodness Todd is the most patient person I know.

The drain is coming out today! I am ecstatic. I feel like I will have my life back. I can start physical therapy or actually, start exercising on my own. I can leave the house without the non zip-up top. And, I'm hopeful that since I will not have to spend time dressing the drain, putting in new bandages, and climbing into my tops, that it won't take me an hour to get ready.

I'm still unsure how pulling clothes on over my head will go. Teaching tomorrow should be interesting. I am so excited to be back at Sculpt Fusion tomorrow morning! I hope I remember how to teach. It feels like a lifetime ago, but it has only been two weeks.

Yesterday was a challenge and a blessing. Kind of like all of these days, I suppose. I'd basically hit the wall with being stuck in the house. I would not be a model prisoner if I were ever incarcerated.

Jannine Oberg, who does Emotional Freedom Technique (EFT) work, came over and did a session with me. EFT is based upon a variety of modalities, utilizing acupressure and meridian work from Chinese medicine. I really liked it. Thank you Jannine!

What resonated with me is that you need to acknowledge and work through the negative emotions, instead of just burying them and trying to "look on the bright side." I've struggled with that concept a lot. I am accustomed to putting on the happy, strong, positive Claire face, no matter what. I am not comfortable in the dark. And, believe me, shadows are obscuring the light. A wise friend told me to accept that you are in the dark at times, but use the "flashlight" into the shadows to find the gifts.

In EFT, you work through the negative or stagnant thoughts and feelings and then make room for the positive. I felt a huge shift when we came to the point where I acknowledged that "CANCER" can have some of my time but, I will not allow "CANCER" to take all my happiness, occupy all my waking thoughts, or take over my world. I will allow "CANCER" part of my attention, but I will also live my life and not allow it to invade every part of it. I take back my recreation, my love, my work, my time for me. So there!

56

Meg put it best: Ding Dong the Drain is Gone, the Wicked Drain...faa laa laa...

Regrettably, the drain is considered bio-hazardous waste and the doctor extinguished all my evil plans for its demise.

So go the best-laid plans.

Seeing as I am such a secretive and mysterious type, I cannot resist sharing some details.

The lovely Meredith accompanied me to the drain-removal party and was lucky enough to watch the festivities from the front row. The doctor quizzed me, ensuring that I was at the acceptable drainage level. I am pleased to say that I didn't have to fudge the numbers at all. And, believe me, over the last week I've been tempted!

First, she had to "milk the drain." This consists of holding onto it with both hands and pulling on it like I was Bessie the cow. Or, back in college playing intramural tug-o-war. Black dots swam before my eyes and the room became very hot. She reclined me back on the table. I'm not sure if that is standard procedure or if she worried I was going to faint. Either way, it helped.

Milking took a while. One tug was so intense that my left leg kicked up involuntarily, like a marionette. Good to know that the right side is connected to the left leg. I hope never to discover if the opposite is true. Meredith later told me that she almost flew to my aid. I guess the milking looked as awful as it felt.

After I was sufficiently "milked," she removed the drain. She then showed me about four inches of tubing that had been inside me, above the sutures. Did I mention that this thing was stitched in to me? Four inches of tube! I almost tossed my cookies at that. It was gross enough seeing the external portion of the drain that hung around for twelve days, much less the interior.

Meredith then took the scenic route from Scripps Hospital along the La Jolla Coast past Torrey Pines Park to the beach. I love that stretch of road: dramatic cliffs, crashing waves, fertile marshland. She then walked me. Wait! No! She did not walk me! I walked myself!!! While wearing a tank top. No jacket required. Amazing!

It has been seven hours. I think it will take a few days for me to feel free.

Tomorrow: teaching. The first step to feeling free.

February 18th: Teaching and Mystery Vegetables
Today was a good day! A great day! An emotional day!

First cry: driving to teach yoga this morning. I was nervous. What if I had forgotten how? Would it feel different?

Then, my nervousness and crying jag were interrupted when some Camry nearly knocked me out of my lane. I screamed at him. Immediately, life returned to status quo. I still get Tourette's when I drive on the Interstate. It was a Thursday morning like any other.

I know it is a contradiction that I teach yoga, advocating calm and peace of mind, but I think my driving issues are primal and deep. It all goes back to my Corsican grand-père. That's my story and I'm sticking to it.

The familiar faces and warm welcome in all of my classes today felt amazing. I am so blessed to be part of this community. I remembered how to teach. I, unfortunately, could not lift my arm above shoulder height or touch my toes. Mind you, I am Gumby and have always been able to just lay my palm flat on the floor. Not today! Humbling. Now, I can truly empathize with all my runner students. I can't wait to get my flexibility back.

I teach in a room heated to 95 degrees, with 40% humidity. Thus, my shirt was soaked. Luckily, my friend April was there to help me peel it off. This was the first time I had put something on over my head. And, lululemon tops ensure that your ta-tas are secure. Just hard to remove when you cannot move your arm or feel your underarm. Again, for a super-independent person who doesn't like to ask for help, this is a journey. I've been dressing myself for years.

Cry #2: My ActiveX peeps brought me flowers. Beautiful flowers: nice job! It was perfect, sunny and breezy outside during our class.

Then, my wonderful family at lululemon Carlsbad is a host site for Garden of Eden, a local, organic farm that provides fresh produce. They were kind enough to donate a shipment to me this week. I am overflowing with veggies and fruit! Fabulous.

Here's the catch: my old nemesis, Kale, (ha hah!) was on top of the vegetables. Luckily, there are two small bunnies that live on my cul-de-sac. I left the special treat out for them. They were very pleased. I bet there will be an extra lift in their hop tomorrow.

The second catch: I didn't know what half of the vegetables were!! Seriously!!

59

Lettuce: check.

Spinach: check.

Oranges, lemons, avocados: check.

Here's where things got sticky:

Mysterious small reddish-purple carrot-looking things--NO idea.

More mysterious reddish-purple carrot-looking things with what looked like chard attached--WHAT?!

Some type of fresh herb--HUH?!

Luckily, Lauren called to educate me. Reddish carrot things are indeed carrots!! Other reddish things are beets, herb is oregano. Who knew? Very excited to try them!

Cry #3: Spoke to Julian today. We had another discussion about chemotherapy and I must admit that he is very convincing. I'm still waiting to see how I feel after meeting with two different oncologists and receiving answers to all of my questions about treatment scenarios. I couldn't stem the tears.

Maybe the doctors will tell me chemo is optional. That would help my dilemma about needing a touch-up for my highlights.

Saturday, February 20th: Speechless...

Tonight rendered me speechless.

For those of you who know me, you'll realize that is a rarity. Okay, okay, it has never happened. In fact, I cannot recall another situation where I didn't have a response. I am humbled. I am blessed. I am the luckiest person I know. I am floating in a haze of warmth and beauty.

Tonight, the lovely and inspirational Kim Stahler, owner of Sculpt Fusion Yoga, the studio where I teach most of my classes, held a Donation yoga class for me. Cancer isn't cheap! Between missing two weeks of teaching because of the surgery and the drain, very expensive health insurance and medical bills, and the uncertainty of how many classes I will miss over the next six months for treatment and appointments, the financial part of this journey is daunting. Tonight was a boon.

I am glowing. The studio looked beautiful. Candles and flowers everywhere. So many people attended, not just students, but people from all areas of my life. My Rescue House peeps. My Frog's students. Some people I didn't even know! Some showed up for the vino part and skipped the Vinyasa. Actually, I guess Todd and I did the same thing! The gifted Maria graciously taught the class this evening.

What rendered me speechless? It began with feisty Jenn Richardson asking everyone to sit in a circle around me. By candlelight, Jenn spoke from the heart and led us in a healing Om circle. She shared a personal story of how I had inspired her and lifted her up when she went through teacher training.

She reciprocated tonight. I cannot recall each word, just the message that everyone loved me, that they were there to support me, to help me, to hold me up, and that everyone visualize me healthy, happy and laughing. The power and beautiful energy in the room blew me away. I had nothing to say.
Did I mention that is a first?

Tonight was yet another affirmation that exiting the corporate rat race to teach yoga full time was the right decision for me. As I've said all along, I am awed at the love and support from those around me including those who are close and those who I don't know that well. My man, my friends, my family, my community. This cancer has reconnected me with people I've missed having in my life and not been in contact with for years.

I'm so happy that I had tonight. Yesterday and most of today were hell. The oncologist shall be described on Monday's entry, after I get a second opinion. I'm not going to ruin the beauty of tonight. Let's just say if I'd written before 6 p.m. or last night, it wouldn't have been pretty.
I love ending on a positive note.

Sunday, February 21st: Still riding last night's high

No sleep again last night. My heart is bursting with gratitude. My brain is operating at warp speed attempting to process everything from my oncology meeting. The second opinion is tomorrow.

This morning was lovely. I attended my first yoga class since surgery with several of the lululemon ladies. We anticipated a restorative class consisting of lying on the floor for an hour or so, snuggled into blankets, supported by bolsters. Yummy. It turned out to be gentle yoga and there were a few down dogs. No down dog for me yet, but I was happy to see that each day the range of motion in my right arm and shoulder improves. I hope to lift it overhead by the end of the week. I am trying to ignore how much it looks and feels like a shark chomped a chunk of my flesh.

On another note, I've been compiling a list of names and numbers of referrals. Specifically, it is a list of other breast cancer survivors similar to me in age and situation. I haven't felt up to calling anyone yet. Until today.

I spoke with an incredible woman from Boulder, Colorado. When I learned that she was 37 when she was diagnosed, after her return from her honeymoon in Kauai (one of my favorite places on earth), that she was a yoga instructor (same studio as one where I teach here) and that she was a rock star seven-year survivor, I wanted to speak with her. I was especially intrigued about how she used her yoga: both teaching and practicing, to stay strong throughout her treatment.

Our discussion was great. What she shared really resonated with me. Her primary point was that you've got one chance to attack the cancer with every tool at your disposal. That time is now. She didn't want to look back and regret not trying everything.

She used complementary care: nutrition, yoga, acupuncture and other holistic methods to keep her strong throughout surgeries, chemotherapy, and radiation. Our discussion helped settle some of the conflicts I've been experiencing regarding conventional chemotherapy treatment. Not that anybody wants chemo, but I didn't believe it would help me at all. My stance is softening. Is this just part of the process?

It is interesting how my views are shifting. Is it acceptance? Resignation? Fear? A lowering of my standards? I've now discussed wigs with more than one person. Wow. Two weeks ago, I couldn't have fathomed it.

Monday, February 22nd: Free Housecleaning!

Too good to be true! Imagine getting free maid service once a month! Someone to take care of those pesky baseboards, toilets and shower doors. It can be yours. Yes, for free. All you need to do is qualify.

Unfortunately, the criterion is chemotherapy.

I qualify. I am going to go through chemotherapy. I've said it. I've written it. It shall come to pass. Wow. I know tons of women have survived and thrived through treatment, but there is still a feeling of how can this be my path? Really? This is going to be three-quarters of 2010.

I am not doing it for the maid service, in case you were curious.

What changed my mind? That there could be cells that broke away from the tumor that are too small to be picked up on any scan. That those cells are waiting to multiply. And, from what I interpreted, if I don't go through the chemo now and wait until later, it may be too late. I get it. I don't like it, but I understand.

I had a lot of plans, dreams and goals for this year. I even made a list on January 1st. On January 2nd, I found the lump. This year is going to be very different than I anticipated. I was looking at this year as the time to truly grow my business, increase my private clientele to a point where I was thriving financially as well as professionally. I was hoping to film for Exercise TV in early spring, which now seems out of the question.

It is frustrating. I feel like my career was blossoming. And, for now, I've got to focus on just maintaining my class schedule, not grow it. For now. It is tough. It is scary financially. I'm scared that I'll lose opportunities. I already have.

On the other hand, I've been blown away by how generous, warm and caring everyone has been. Who knows if I'd ever experience this level of support otherwise? I knew that my immediate circle would be fantastic; that is why I have them in my life. But, those who I'm getting closer to due to this illness have shown me such unconditional support. An incredible silver lining.

I must share my two oncology appointments. Friday consisted of an absolutely brutal three-plus-hours meeting with my oncologist. Today, I went in for a second opinion. Both doctors gave me basically the same information. Apparently, breast cancer is so common that there is a computer program where they can plug in age, tumor size, grade, and spread and spit out a treatment protocol. Is this the epidemic of our lifetime?

Recipe: Six Rounds of Chemo every three weeks. T (Taxotere) A(Adriamycin) C(Cytoxan.) Or, the second doctor suggested just TC. Seven weeks of Radiation. Five Days a Week. And, la piece de resistance: Five YEARS of Tamoxifin. All of these ingredients impart a proliferation of side effects ranging from mildly annoying to traumatic to monstrous.

I'm already exhausted from the appointments, the tests, the phone calls, the waiting, and the driving. Not to mention the pain I continue to experience. And, the hunger. Tomorrow's CT Scan requires six hours of fasting. Friday's surgery also requires me to starve myself. My car shall be slinking into the drive-thru at In-N-Out soon.

This has been the longest seven weeks of my life. Seven months loom ahead of me like an insurmountable mountain with no peak in sight. I'll take some yogic wisdom and do my best to live in the present moment. And, try to remember that cancer is just part of my life. It cannot be all of it.

Wednesday, February 24th: Spot on my Liver

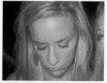

I love all the comments. Jessie--I like the idea of nine months of gestation to baby Claire. I was rather pleased with me pre-rebirth, but why not?

Warning: I am simmering with negativity and I'm about to erupt. Despite the unbearable pressure, a little light remains inside the lava pit that is my emotional core. Gratitude first.

I am very happy that my dad, brother and sister are in town to see me. We've had a great visit so far. It was a beautiful day and we went to La Jolla. We also went to lululemon so they could see what lululemon is, what it stands for in the community and my life and, most importantly, where my photo would be on the wall. It was wonderful to be able to share that part of my life with them.

We also ate yummy meals at Georges at the Cove and Third Corner, respectively.

Now: the dark. So, my oncologist phoned me today. Personally. Mind you, I receive almost daily calls from Scripps for scheduling, test results and the like. Today, my oncologist picked up the phone herself and dialed my digits. This is not a good sign.

A little background: yesterday was a blur of poking, prodding and starving. The Breast Cancer Gene test where they sucked out what felt like the rest of my blood. A Chest X-Ray, not so bad. A CT and PET Scan that were a nightmare.

My friend Zoe accompanied me and was planning to stay with me. Well, they kicked her out. Here's the scoop: the technician takes you into a room, sits you in a chair, and injects a radioactive isotope with dye into your arm. Then, any possible activity is forbidden. I could not read. I could not talk on the phone. I could not move. I had to sit, completely still, in a chair with this IV sticking out of my arm for 45 minutes. Well, you can only imagine how the mind wanders. I could not suppress thoughts of my late brother Andre, a hemophiliac, who spent about a day per month in the hospital for all of his 33 years. How did he endure it?

I sobbed unabashedly. Alone. For 45 minutes.

Next, I was stuffed into the coffin-like machine for the two scans. The first one is feet first and the second is head first. Again, you are completely immobilized.

Insult to injury: You have to fast for six hours. At this rate of starvation, I will look anorexic enough to sashay down a Paris runway. When I am deprived of food for more than a few hours, it is not pretty. Luckily, Zoe is a saint and after she was unceremoniously kicked out, she went and bought me lunch. Including a big chocolate donut. Cancer-loving sugar be damned. After shoveling in all of the healthy stuff and the donut I felt almost human. Almost.

Now for the bad news: My doctor called to tell me that the CT/PET results worried not only her, but two radiologists as well. There is a 9mm spot on my liver. She said that at first she wasn't worried, that it looked subtle to her and could be a birthmark or something benign. But after the second radiologist read it and also expressed concern, they want to do a super-special MRI of my abdomen with Eovist?? Whatever that might be.

She called me because she didn't want to wait until our appointment on the 8th and lose another week. Treatment apparently will be very different if this liver issue is cancer. The liver is the first place where anything metastasizes. All I can think about is all that beer and grain alcohol at University of Virginia. Did I have one jello shot too many 20 years ago?

During our conversation, I informed her that I agreed to do chemo. She asked what days worked for me and I told her Fridays, so I could recuperate over the weekend and minimize my time away from teaching. Teaching helps me maintain a shred of sanity. She said she'd get it scheduled and we should start my first round on the 12th of March. That is, unless this liver spot dictates otherwise.

Each time I accept or resign myself to this nightmare; it gets worse. I finally process all the information on chemotherapy and agree to it. Now, possible metastasizing to the liver? I don't know how much longer I can keep it together. Where will this end? What the hell will they want to do if it is in my liver? How strong am I supposed to be?

Maybe it is time to sell my car and travel and just enjoy how I feel now, for however long it lasts. The idea tempts me. Todd? Jake and Oreo? Anyone?

Friday, February 26th: Nobody puts baby in the corner

Remember that line? Prior to my latest surgical adventure, there was an operating room back-up. The pre-op nurse brought me back to the launching pad area and was then informed that I was second in line for surgery. Oops. I was placed in the back corner of the huge area and curtains drawn around me. An IV was inserted into my hand in order to begin giving me fluids. Thank goodness because I was more dehydrated than I was after visiting Amsterdam in college.

The nurse told me not to feel rejected for being in second place and that they'd get to me after about 45 minutes. As I lay semi-hallucinating on my gurney, I kept thinking of Patrick Swayze's infamous line in Dirty Dancing, "Nobody puts baby in the corner." Very strange to be rolled toward surgery and then placed into a holding pattern.

I love my surgeon. She is amazing: cute, funny, warm, caring. I feel very comfortable with her. When I told her about the liver spot, she reassured me that Dr. K, my oncologist, would have notified her if she was really concerned. What a relief. Even with my family and teaching distracting me, the last few days have been shaky. This liver spot issue scares me. It has to be a birthmark or a false positive. It must.

It was very therapeutic having my family here for a few days. We enjoyed some good food, wine and the San Diego sunshine. They headed home this morning.

After they departed, I taught my Frogs yoga class. Teaching really is helping me maintain a sliver of composure. When I teach I am fully present and not thinking about tests, cancer and this surreal nightmare. I had a special blessing: visitors from my past came all the way to San Diego to take my class. Connie grew up right down the street from me in Virginia. We reconnected on Facebook and voila. Thank you Connie!

Maybe I've turned a corner. I woke up feeling fine. I feel okay now. Methinks I'm a little buzzed from my Vicodin, but that is okay! No drain, no pain, no trauma.

My wonderful man Todd drove me through In-N-Out and I had my first cheeseburger in almost two months. I've had no meat. I don't think one fantastic, mouth-watering cheeseburger will kill me. Tomorrow it is back to the pure organic, super green regime. I will get an Emerald Bliss. With Wheat Grass. I promise.

Saturday, February 27th: Stay Ahead of the Pain Meds!

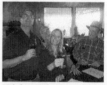

This photo is from Leonesse Winery. It captures my family dynamic quite well: My brother Robert, my sister Yael, yours truly and my dad laughing at us all. We visited Temecula for the afternoon so I could really get a head start on my pain medication prior to the surgery yesterday. There's nothing like a little red wine to get through surgery eve.

The recovery from this second surgery is significantly better than the first. No drain. No terrible fear at the potential of chemotherapy. Over the last few weeks, the chemotherapy became my reality. Wow. I started to do some more research in my natural medicine book on the antioxidants, vitamins and nutrition to counterbalance the poisonous drugs soon to be injected into my system. My brain is full.

I read about the side-effects again and it is unfathomable what will transpire over the next four months. Then, seven weeks of radiation. No, no, no! Simply enumerating the supplements I should take is overwhelming: the fish oil, the enzymes, the greens, the juicing, and the vitamins. What will help strengthen the white blood cells, which supplements will help diminish the bone marrow damage? It is enough to push me over the brink.

Then, I received the first bill from my insurance company. Thousands of dollars, and it is just for January. No surgeries yet, none of these recent fancy scans and tests included. The financial aspect of this is daunting. Despite having good insurance, I know that the price of poison isn't cheap. And, my COBRA coverage ends in August, right in the middle of radiation. I sure hope that I can get it extended.

I'm a whiner today, aren't I? It was a tough week. The liver spot threw me for a loop. I felt fine but the minute I started writing, the fears emerged. I've got several yucky tests over the next weeks, including a four-hour bone scan, the MRI with Eovist for the liver and an EKG. Whew.

Okay, shift gears Claire: I am very grateful for my family's visit and love, for Todd (who insists that I give him photographer credit for this photo), for all of my awesome friends' support. My lovely girls are taking me to Palm Springs next weekend so that I can finally get my craving for lazing by the pool fulfilled. I cannot wait to just absorb some sunshine, read a book, and escape for a little while.

Time for pain meds: they tell you not to fall behind or they won't work! God forbid.

Sunday, February 28th: Big Tree Fall Hard

Another favorite movie line: this time from Wedding Crashers. Well, today I walked in Vince Vaughn's shoes. I was tackled out of left field.

As I've mentioned, this second surgery was a piece of cake compared to the first. I'm taking the pain medication as directed, which may be why I'm challenged to construct a coherent sentence. I suppose that because the second surgery didn't come with the drain from hell that it doesn't feel as traumatic? My arm continues to heal, which helps.

It was a beautiful, sunny day and Todd and I went to the lagoon for a walk. Not a "time to walk the Claire," rather a walk together at our old pace. It felt lovely and almost normal.

Then, voluntarily, I requested Todd stop at Jimbo's to buy me an Emerald Bliss. The taste fails to improve. Eternal optimist that I am, I continue to hope each time that I'll take a sip and won't gag. Nope. This bitter brew better be magic! I must admit to feeling smug and virtuous. Obviously, as I feel compelled to report it in my blog each time I drink one.

When we arrived home, I was feeling fired up and vacuumed. Then, I selected two workout DVDs that I usually find easy. I need to exercise! I detest feeling the muscles in my legs, arms and core just atrophying away.

Skinny-fat. Repulsive. As I was about to start one of the DVDs, a wave of tiredness and nausea floored me.

No option existed except to lie down. Two hours later, I swam back into consciousness. Was this from the pain medication? I guess I did just have surgery less than 48 hours ago and need to take it slowly. But I felt so great earlier!

Is this foreshadowing? Is this what will happen during treatment? I'll feel great and then all of a sudden crash? Without warning or control? No option but to lie down or fall over? I couldn't help sobbing when I woke up. I've always considered myself so strong and cannot seem to remember that feeling.

This battle isn't day by day. It is hour by hour.

Chapter 3: March

Monday, March 1ˢᵗ: Pranayama and the Contrast MRI

Pranayama is one of the most important concepts in yoga. Breath keeps us in the present moment. Breath connects our body to our mind and to our spirit. Today, it was the most important concept in my dye-contrast MRI. Who knew?

What is Pranayama? For those who aren't familiar with the term, here are a few definitions:

According to Patanjali's Yoga Sutras, "Regulation of breath or the control of prana is the stoppage of inhalation and exhalation, which follows after securing that steadiness of posture or seat, asana.

Technical Definition ahead: Pranayama is breath control. Proper breathing and awareness of the breath is very important. Swami Yogananda says, "Breath is the cord that ties the soul to the body."

Your breathing directly affects the mental states. Breathing exercises help to control bodily functions. A regular, deep breath enables one to feel calm and an irregular breath can make you feel anxious. Yoga Breathing helps to re-charge the cells in the body and re-energizes the brain cells; thus, the body is rejuvenated.

Hopefully, some of that resonates.

How does this apply to the MRI today? It started the same way as the others.

Change into an unattractive gown: check.

Layer another gown on top of it: check.

Notice how much more attractive the Ugg boots look compared to the running shoes and socks worn during the Breast MRI: check.

Helpful technician inserted yet another dye-filled IV into my left arm. Same technician astutely noted that it looked like my left arm "had been getting some action." Um, yeah.

Get strapped onto the bed. Choose Alternative Rock for my headphones. Although the MRI clanging drowns out most of the music, I did enjoy half a Foo Fighters song and that makes me happy. Get inserted into the coffin-like machine.

Here's where the Pranayama comes in. The test consisted of being instructed to start and stop my breath. Several times, he told me to hold my breath for very long periods.

A few times I wasn't sure if I was still holding it, sometimes I thought I'd faint before I heard his voice telling me to breathe. I'm used to teaching breath work, studying it, and using it and I could barely hold my breath long enough. Is this how some of my students feel when I continually tell them to inhale and exhale? If so, I'm sorry!

Did I have any epiphanies while I practiced my breath work? Nope. Just a series of random thoughts: How do bigger people fit in here? If I stick my tongue out could I lick the top? How would a smoker hold his or her breath long enough? How many more times will I have to hold my breath? What if I pass out in here? Should I have selected Guns-n-Roses instead of alternative rock? What will I have for breakfast when I'm hatched from the machine? Not exactly profound.

And, the elephant in the room: will this test reveal that the spot on my liver is benign?

Wednesday, March 3rd: Radioactive bone scans and wig shopping

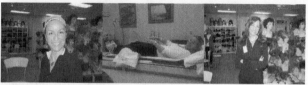

Whew, the last few days have been an absolute whirlwind of tests, teaching, brow shaping, registering for the cancer yoga therapy training at Prana Yoga, and wig shopping with the girls.

For the bone scan yesterday, yet another radioactive isotope was injected into my abused flesh. Although they continue to assure me that there are no lasting effects of the isotopes, they did inquire whether I was traveling or going to a federal building in the next few days. Just in case.

For some reason, after I reclined on the conveyor belt, Edgar the technician taped my feet together. Very odd. He flipped the switch and presto, I was rolling toward the machine. The top was very low and I felt certain that it would shave off the tip of my nose. Edgar assured me that it would not. Remember the old-fashioned magic shows where they insert the "assistant" into a box? Or, the old movies where the villain ties the helpless female to the railroad tracks? Both scenarios fit. I did emerge with my nose intact.

Teaching has been amazing this week. My yoga and Pilates students rock and I am grateful to have the opportunity to teach. I truly don't think I'd remain sane without it. Sanity being a relative term.

On the subject of teaching, I registered today to take a two-weekend workshop: Yoga for Cancer Therapy. Yes, I am taking it the weekend of March 19th and the weekend of April 2nd. Yes, I shall have my second chemo treatment on the 2nd. What better place for me to be that weekend than surrounded by healers? I can be the real-time guinea pig for how yoga can help. I feel that the training will be invaluable for me personally and who knows? I may end up using this training and journey to help others have an easier time.

After registering, I headed down to the wig store to meet April and Lauren. Although I wanted this to be fun, I ended up feeling nauseous and not just because the wig store is next to Hooters. I think the radioactive injections are getting to me.

Trying on the wigs made me feel like I was sporting an animal on my head. The best ones are human hair and cost upwards of $700. Yes, SEVEN HUNDRED DOLLARS. Fifteen percent medical discount. It didn't feel as playful and fun as I had hoped. It was overwhelming.

The styles that were okay length and cut-wise weren't available in the color I wanted. I'm very visual so it was tough for me to picture the hair in the right color. The one wig that seemed okay was only in Marble Brown. See photo above. I can order it in Golden Wheat (with a $300 deposit) but I only got to see a swatch of it. Kind of like when you go to Home Depot and buy paint based on a miniscule paint square. This is how our bedroom ended up sky blue instead of eggshell.

What did I learn today? I love my friends: thank you girls for your honesty, support and humor!

We established that I am never to have short hair. Especially a short bob. Ever. Even Veronica, the wig fitter ripped it off my head and ran to get a long one. Notice the lack of photographic evidence here.

I just don't know if I can do it. Frankly, I thought I looked better with the skull cap then any of the wigs. I'm going to go see a few women who do this specifically for cancer treatment: they hand sew them to fit, trim them, thin them, etc.

Maybe it won't feel so weird.

Can we call "Cut?" I quit as star of this movie.

Thursday, March 4th: Shades of gray

Good news first: The Breast Cancer Gene test came back negative. Yay. No double mastectomy or ovary removal in my immediate future.

Not so good news: Or, shall I say inconclusive news. The MRI results for the liver spot are in. My doctor called me and the MRI showed a 6mm spot (tiny) on my liver, confirming the CT and PET scan from last week.

Unfortunately, nobody knows what it is. Her gut tells her that it isn't anything serious but she cannot confirm that. She's been doing this a long time and I trust her judgment.

Worst case scenario: if it is the cancer spreading to my liver that means it is "incurable." They can still do treatment, but they can never pronounce me "cured." Not quite sure what that means: a lifetime of gray area?

So, the head of radiology wants to do ANOTHER CT scan of my liver. Yes, the horrible one that requires six hours of fasting, a radioactive isotope and no movement for 45 minutes. He will do it personally and analyze it as we go. If he sees something on it real-time, he will do a biopsy. The problem is that the spot is so small, they aren't sure if they can biopsy it. The thought of a needle going into my liver for a biopsy chills me to the bone.

There is a one-in-three shot of the spot being visible and thus biopsy-able (making up a word and I don't care) and my doctor thinks that I should try. At least we'd have an answer if it is a birthmark or a benign cyst. If they can't tell, we are just going to have to treat it as regular breast cancer as planned and keep checking back to see if it grows. If it grows, then it is cancer.

I'm choosing to believe it is a birthmark. I'll have the additional test next week, but we will stay with the plan of starting chemotherapy on Thursday the 11th. Part of me wants to skip the test. It sucked last time. I am digging deep on the vocabulary today.

I'm absolutely, completely exhausted. Toast. I've lost track of the tests, appointments, injections and phone calls. I'm so thrilled that I've got no appointments tomorrow and will spend the weekend in Palm Springs. Three blissful days without having to be anywhere at a certain time seems like heaven. I have the best friends ever. And, not just because they take me places.

Must sleep. Must recharge.

Friday, March 5th: Cowardly spot

I'm so excited for the girls' trip to the desert tomorrow. Escape with three amazing, strong, beautiful women. I don't care if it rains and we end up sitting on the couch drinking champagne and eating bon-bons, oops, I mean eating kale patties. Chased with wheatgrass shots.

Today was 90 percent excellent. 10 percent rough.

The Excellent: sleeping in late with my boyfriend for the first time that I can recall in recent history. It was a lovely, relaxing morning.

Meeting my friend Nikki for breakfast at St. Tropez, one of my favorite places on earth for breakfast. She is rocking her new life in Hollywood and I'm so proud and happy for her! When she is a famous movie actress, she will bring Robert Pattinson to me. Go Team Edward.

Taught my lovely 10:35 a.m. Frogs Encinitas yoga class. Love these people!! Such great energy. Then, I had a true workout afterwards in the Pilates studio. It felt wonderful to have a full-body workout and feel my upper body strength beginning to return. One of the Pilates students left me a moving card and a bamboo, comfy throw that is the softest thing I've ever felt. Thank you Lori for the kind words (although some who've known me longer might question you describing me as wholesome and innocent but I'll take it!) I will bring my blankie to chemo for sure!

Next stop, lululemon Carlsbad for a little retail therapy, ambassador style. Wonderful people, bright colors, fun styles and a pair of perfect comfy soft sweatpants. I felt awesome when I left. Thank you fabulous lululemon team! The photo proofs arrive in the next few days. I can't wait to see them.

The Rough: So, a beautiful day, right? Well, the 10 percent was awful. It is that pesky liver spot. Dratted liver spot. Begone liver spot. Or, at least stand up and identify yourself as a birthmark for goodness sake. PET, CT and MRI and you still won't admit you are a mole or birthmark. Coward.

Scripps called to schedule my liver biopsy for Tuesday afternoon. All afternoon. Check in at 1 p.m. for blood work. Procedure at 3 p.m. Sedation, as they are going to biopsy the liver. That is, they will if they can discern it on the ultrasound/CT scan. My fear is that I'll spend the whole day there and they still won't be able to identify it or biopsy it.

Now I can't teach my yoga class Tuesday night or my Pilates class Wednesday morning, just in case the sedation is still affecting me on Wednesday morning.

Simply put, it feels like more lost time that I'll never get back. I hate missing out on my life. Even though these tests are now part of my life, I just don't want it to be all of my life. Four days of next week are booked with appointments and tests and the crowning glory: chemo.

Tomorrow is vacation! Nothing to do but relax and have fun for 48 whole hours. Bring it on!

Sunday, March 7th: A beautiful respite...

Sunday night of the "big" week. I'm starting to completely, totally freak out about starting chemotherapy this week. I've compiled my seemingly endless list of natural supplements to buy prior to starting so I can enhance the positive effects and help negate the rest. It is really, really long. And not a little overwhelming. I want a rewind. I don't want this week to start.

This weekend was perfect. Lissa and Kirsten treated me to a relaxing, fun, girly time. The drive out to the desert was easy and we rejoiced whenever the temperature gauge in the car inched up another degree. We pulled up to the Viceroy and entered the modern doorway into our magical weekend kingdom.

Our room was beautiful, very retro-hip, with a South of France feel. Fashionista Kirsten taught me how to tie a sarong and although it was complicated for me, I think I got it right. Multi-talented Lissa played bartender, stirring up the requisite fruity drinks to enjoy by the pool. We sashayed out the sliding doors directly to the pool. My fantasy of reclining by the pool with a fruity drink was fulfilled.

Laughter, sunshine, warmth, good friends: recipe for complete relaxation. We didn't pretend that the cancer didn't exist but for the weekend, it stayed in the background.

After a wonderful Red Carpet Facial (I am watching the Oscars on the couch with Todd and Jake after all), we enjoyed the late afternoon and got ready for what would be a very entertaining evening. Lissa, yes, the multitalented one also happens to be a make-up artist, hair stylist and photographer. Lucky Kirsten and me! We sat on the bathroom floor with our champagne and got beautiful. It felt like we were back in school: I forgot how much fun it can be to just spend hours with the girls, being girls. You know, back when you'd have so much fun getting ready, anticipating the night ahead and nine times out of 10, it was the best part of the night.

The rest of the night lived up to the primping. We stayed within the walls of our magic Viceroy kingdom and headed to the lobby bar. We never had to leave our stools and were entertained for the rest of the evening. Yummy drinks, tasty food, colorful local characters and more good conversation. As evidenced by the photos!

We closed the evening back in the room and laid our pampered heads on the pillows, slumbering before the clock struck midnight. A perfect day.

We returned this morning after a tasty breakfast, poolside.

From the bottom of my heart, thank you ladies for this escape. I haven't felt this relaxed in more than two months. I'll try to return to the feeling over and over as the future unfolds.

Monday, March 8th: Five-Finger Forehead

Day One of an interminable week is winding down. Appointment with Dr. K to discuss the next 18 weeks of treatment. We set up all of the dates and that gives me a small measure of relief. Or control. Or, shall I say, apparent control.

Three more vials of blood sucked out accompanied by yet another ode to my beautiful veins. Apparently, I am the dream destination for any needle or IV. Big, healthy veins. Who knew they'd become such an attribute?

Met with the fantastic Patti at her home salon and selected my new hair. She was so sweet, clever and helpful. Her specialty is working with cancer patients and she made my day. She'll customize the wig, making the hairline natural and give me the gift of not looking too different.

Also, we made a startling discovery: I don't have an abnormally large head after all! My head circumference is actually a little smaller than average although my forehead is bigger. Much bigger. I have a Five-finger Forehead as opposed to the normal Three-finger Forehead.

We also ordered hat hair that is designed to go under a baseball cap or hat and be cooler and super-realistic looking. I think that I'll be going the scarf route for teaching yoga. Now, I need to find some cool Hawaiian print scarves and learn how to tie them. Don't have a clue...I also need some assistance hat shopping!

I left Patti's feeling a little lighter. What a blessing.

Three days until the first "C" treatment. My dance card remains filled with appointments. I'm not going to list out the rest of the appointments leading up to 8 a.m. Thursday morning. I'm going to practice taking this day by day.

Tuesday is liver biopsy. Maybe. If the head of Interventional Radiology can find the teeny liver spot on the CT scan, he will attempt the biopsy. I hope that he can't see it because I really am dreading them digging into my liver. My friend Angie is coming down from Hollywood to take me to the hospital and I hope we get to leave early, go for a hike and eat a yummy dinner instead. A girl can dream.

What started out as a challenging Monday ended on a positive note with Todd cooking me a healthy, delicious dinner. Even though he is in trouble for not finishing his broccoli.

Wednesday, March 10th: Chemo-Eve

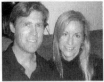

Shiny new Tang-orange lululemon bag packed:
Bamboo soft throw to snuggle into: check
New *In Touch* and *In Style* magazines: check
March by Geraldine Brooks: check
IPod and IPod with movies: check
Earphones (almost forgot!): check

Chemotherapy at 8 a.m. sharp tomorrow. Pre-chemotherapy acupuncture at 7 a.m. I've been trying not to freak out all day, but it has been a challenge. The first dosage of steroids did not enhance my usual angelic patience while sitting in traffic on Interstate 5 this morning. Compounding my stress: the liver biopsy yesterday may go down in history as the worst procedure to date.

Residual pain and nausea lingered from the "twilight" sedation and Vicodin and the needles that entered into my right lower rib cage. The Amazing Angie drove down after training her clients in Hollywood to take me to the hospital. We left at 12:30. Admittance, more blood work, entry into a shared room with curtains between the patients. The doctor was supposed to do the procedure at 3 p.m. but didn't come to my partition until 4:22. So, I lay there in the bed, with an IV in my arm for over two hours waiting.

When he finally arrived, he approached the man across the way saying hello to Mr. Petretti. Way to instill confidence in me: if he couldn't read my name on the chart, how the hell was he going to locate the spot on my liver? I was yelling "Over here, Ms. Petretti over here!!"

Finally, the nurse got him and we got down to business. He confirmed Dr. K's concerns that if he couldn't discern the spot on the CT scan we couldn't do the biopsy. I informed him that I was visualizing that as the case and that I'd prefer to skip the biopsy, thank you very much. I would be thrilled to leave prior to him sampling some of my liver. Liver, liver, liver. With fava beans and a fine Chianti. I need to banish that visual!

I was wheeled in for the CT scan without sedation. Ah, the novelty. No, my feet were not taped together like in the bone scan. No, my boobs did not have slots in which to rest. No, I wasn't injected with radioactive isotopes or dye. So far, so good.

Instead, I was face down with my arms overhead. It was painful due to the second lumpectomy 11 days ago. And, the lymph node incision. And, my artificial disc in my neck. To add insult to injury, the nurse stuffed little plastic tubes of oxygen up my nose. The piece de resistance was taping together my wrists over my head with an ace bandage. As I glanced over at the tech team, two nurses and the doctor were peering at me from behind a big glass window; let's just say I felt a little odd.

Oh yes, they instructed me to make sure not to move. Ummm, how would I? In addition to the above-referenced bondage, they also had a strap over my legs. Again, liver with fava beans and a fine Chianti.

Dr. N informed me that he could do the biopsy. Bring on the twilight sedation. Not full anesthesia but apparently it gives you amnesia. I haven't forgotten the indignities of the position but I don't recall him sticking the biopsy needle into my back four times and taking small pieces of my precious LIVER out. I definitely felt it. And, I still can. My reward for remaining immobile was two Vicodin. And, I wonder why I've felt sick and terrible all day? The biopsy spot is excruciating.

No, we don't have the results yet. Dr. K told the path lab to page her when they arrive. I spoke to her today and I think she is incredible. Whoever told me that she was kind of "stern" missed out because she told me a semi-racy joke today. Hilarious. Maybe she feels comfortable with me. I trust her implicitly, which feels good on chemo eve.

I also had my post-op appointment and the margins were clear on the second lumpectomy so I don't see the surgical team for six months! Yay, my dance card is emptying out. If I just have to go to chemo every three weeks, it will seem like heaven. I deserve my own reserved parking spot at Scripps after the last few months. I've literally been there almost every single day. How refreshing to have some time to myself again.

Let's see: positive and silver lining. Well, I was thrilled to receive the proofs from my lululemon ambassador shoot. Yippee! Shooting at the break of dawn was definitely worth it. The light, the sky, the setting, and the colors all turned out beautifully. It was a wonderful distraction yesterday to pore over the pictures. I look strong and healthy in all the photos. And my hair doesn't look half bad either. HA!

Also, I continue to feel humbled and grateful for the continued support from everyone. Please keep it coming. Believe it or not, I think I'm only just scratching the surface. I think chemo will be a breeze after all the tests but I'm not eager to encounter fatigue, nausea and my big bald head. I am going to teach as much as I can and I am going to get through this. June 24th is the last chemo date. Bring it on!

Thursday, March 11th: Chemo Infusion One... Five to Go

I was amped up this morning. After a sleepless night, I stayed unnaturally high from the steroids and compounded it by taking two more prior to leaving. Luckily, I headed to acupuncture before the hospital.

Lois used acupuncture to help lower my stress level and to temper the nausea I was already experiencing. It worked! I left her office transformed. Todd immediately remarked how my face had calmed down.

Upon arrival, I settled into my recliner and snuggled into my bamboo throw. My chemo nurse's name is Margarita. Like the drink. She is awesome. She explained what was going to transpire for treatment, reviewed potential side effects, and made recommendations for how to handle them. She included a few tidbits I didn't care for: no more manicure/pedicure through chemo because of putting feet in the tubs and possibility for infection. NO! What if I bring my own sterilizer? How will the toes survive?

Back to the skinny on chemo treatment #1. We started with the "A" drug, known as the Red Devil due to its scarlet color and ability to burn flesh on contact. She set up the IV and had to administer it manually through the tube because it is important not to let it flow too quickly. Drug "A" comes with a popsicle to keep the mouth cool. Note the photo: magazine, popsicle, iPod, *Twilight* journal for notes. I was all set. Not bad.

Drug 2 was "C"; the nurse walked away and allowed it to flow into my veins for an hour. It was fine. Compared to the other tests, like the MRIs and liver biopsy, it was a piece of cake. So far, so good.

Before I forget: got the results on the liver biopsy. Surprise, surprise: it was "non-diagnostic" meaning that they cannot determine from the biopsied tissue whether it is cancer or not. Non-conclusive. CT and PET scan, MRI with Eovist, liver biopsy and nothing. So, now we'll just track it on CT scan to see if it grows. I wish I'd just told them to skip that liver biopsy. I'm sure it is nothing.

By this point, I was getting cocky and sending off texts and emails about how much easier chemo was than what I've already endured. Oops.

The minute she started Drug #3, the Taxotere (T), I immediately felt my temperature escalate, saw spots swim before my eyes, and began to suffocate as my throat started closing up. Imagine your throat sealing from the inside out. Luckily, she swiftly stopped it, changed the drip to Benadryl, and followed that with a clear saline. This fun detour added another forty 40 minutes to the treatment. I sure hope that doesn't happen again.

I've got a dizzying assortment of anti-nausea drugs. The co-pay cost $87 for the three-day dosage. Times six. Crazy that is all the insurance covers on it because it is a new drug.

I felt tired. We went to Swamis Café for an acai bowl, which was yummy. When we finally got home, I laid down for a nap for a few hours. When I awoke, my legs were wobbly and tentative as a newborn colt. But, okay. Our first dinner delivery from Marianne arrived. Wow! It was delicious: fresh pasta with tomatoes, mozzarella, basil, balsamic, complemented by spinach salad and sinful brownies. Yum!

Right now, I am sleepy and my stomach is a little jumpy. Not too bad.

Tomorrow, I return for the Neulasta shot. I may do acupuncture again to deal with the nervous belly.

I'm glad it is over and now I know what to expect, at least for the treatments. How the next few days will unfold remains a mystery. I'm approaching it with optimism. I will get through this with flying colors. Yes.
I received two wonderful gifts in the mail: beautiful flowers from my little sis Sue and a Slanket, which looks like a big pink Snuggie. I love it!! Who sent it? There was no card. G'night.

Friday, March 12th: Après-Chemo Day One
Nothing dramatic occurred today. Yippee. Now, I've heard that the first 24 hours aren't bad and if you are going to be hit by some fatigue or pain, it starts on days two through four. We'll see. I'm optimistic that I'll breeze through.

I did feel a bit nauseous when I woke up and took my steroids and the E-nausea drug. I skipped my usual cup of coffee for some green tea. After a shower, Todd walked me around the neighborhood for 22 minutes. It felt great to be outside in the fresh air. I amble like a wobbly colt, but it was nice to move. So far, so good.

Then, I headed in for a session of acupuncture prior to receiving my Neulasta shot. Once again, Lois managed to calm my stomach down in a matter of minutes. She also added a needle that is supposed to help with the negative impact on the white blood cell counts from the chemo drugs. This acupuncture is going to be my saving grace.

The Neulasta shot was sharp but short. Margarita said that possible side effects of the shot include bone pain. Let's hope I skip that. I do have enough Vicodin to supply a major Hollywood party, just in case.

More of my mundane little day: To CVS to pick up my thermometer as I now need to monitor my temperature daily. If it exceeds 100.5, I need to call the doctor. Tea tree oil for my finger nails, which may change color. I'm not sure what that means. Will they turn black? Or green?

I prefer Mademoiselle Pink by Essie. Heavy duty moisturizer to prevent the dryness and possible flakiness that may arise. Finally, a big bottle of Biotene Dry Mouth rinse because all three drugs cause dry mouth, which can result in mouth sores and stomatitis. Yes, let us avoid that. Apparently, you can't get any dental work during chemotherapy treatment either. Oh, the details.

Took a nap and Todd made me get up for Walk Two. This one was about 15 minutes but, definitely a good idea. Next up: dinner. Leftovers from our delicious meal from last night: Marianne: you rock! I do feel a bit queasy and took another anti-nausea pill. (not related to dinner!!)

So, saying that the day after my first chemotherapy was uneventful must be considered a success. I consider it a victory. I'm planning on getting up and going to Rescue House for my cat volunteering session. Always great therapy! Tomorrow will be better.

Thanks for all the great comments. You guys are keeping me lifted up on a cloud of light and love. I'm so blessed and grateful.

Saturday, March 13th: Après-chemo Day Two...

Rolling a little bit slowly, but rolling along nonetheless. Today was the final day of the "E" drug for nausea. I think the nausea wagon is closing its doors this evening. It really hasn't been bad at all. Two analogies for you: hangover or very mild flu.

I whiled away a happy morning at the Rescue House Cat Adoption center at Petco Encinitas. Two fun-filled hours playing with the kitties, snuggling, cleaning up and feeding them. It is so relaxing for me. Again, that joy of doing something that has nothing to do with me and only helps the cats was a lovely way to start my weekend.

I must confess I needed a nap post-cat house, but that is okay. The nap was followed by a walk on the beach with my man. Ocean air is a cure-all. I'm definitely keeping up on the daily walks post-treatment. Not exactly a workout, but it feels like it is helping move these medicines through my system faster. Faster is better. Faster means that when Monday morning dawns, I'll pop out of bed and be ready to go.

Or, slink out of bed. Semantics.

That's all I've got. I'm tired and my head is hurting a bit. Time to go to bed and Spring Forward! More sunshine. Love it.

Sunday, March 14th: Après-chemo Day Three: Beautiful San Diego

What an amazing day in San Diego!

Lissa picked me up and took me for a walk with Maxwell, her perfect, handsome, big, black dog. We went to one of my favorite spots, the Batiquitos Lagoon. It is a verdant green sanctuary with subtle breezes, breathtaking views of pelicans, egrets, ducks and the water. And best of all, a veritable parade of dogs on their Sunday strolls. Fabulous. For both Maxwell and us!

All that fresh air stirred up an appetite. For some reason, I very specifically craved spaghetti with meat sauce and salad. Interesting that I am craving red meat as I cannot recall the last time I had it. Maybe my red blood cells are crying out for some iron? I really want my Dad's spaghetti. He makes the best! Success: Todd and I made the above-referenced wonderful dinner and ate every bite.

Washing my hair today was an odd experience. For some reason, my hair, my teeth and my skin feel weird. I was kind of expecting a chunk of hair to come out in my hands as I was shampooing. I am trying to prevent my mind from wandering in that direction. I plan on having my girls on SOS emergency dial when that chunk emerges. I know it will be time to run to Patti's for my wig. I predict that I will freak out.

Who am I kidding? I know that I will freak out. I feel like I've got a handle right now. The minute my baby fine strands exit stage left...well, the howl will be heard around the globe. And, for those of you familiar with the power of these vocal chords, that is not an exaggeration.

We'll see.

I am hoping that the worst is behind me and that all of the horrid tests, scans, surgeries, pokes, pulls, tugs, hog-tying and indignities of the last few months are over. Five more chemo "infusions." April 1, April 22, May 13, June 3 and June 24. I'm ready to be done.

I have a trip to Australia to plan after all this time-consuming cancer business.

Tuesday, March 16th: Spoke a little too soon...

You know sometimes when something seems too good to be true?

I must admit that I was feeling a bit virtuous this weekend at how well I was handling my first chemotherapy. Perhaps I was even a little self-righteous. Look at me: I'm eating right, I'm doing acupuncture, I'm going on walks and I don't feel too bad. Side-effects: piece of cake. I can handle this, no problem. Laa-dee-daaa.

Well, that didn't last. Sunday evening came crashing down around my ears in the form of a big fat Bone Pain Bat over the head. Whoever named it something as innocuous as Bone Pain should be punished. Must create a new name.

A more accurate description: jaws of death gripping the back of the skull and pulverizing said skull into dust. Slow, inexorable crushing of the bones in a vice. Does anyone recall that scene with Joe Pesci from Goodfellas? Every single bone being crunched between pliers. Not just a "bone" but I'm talking the back of the skull, each vertebra, every tiny bone...throughout my entire body.

Now, I do recall my sister telling me that she'd experienced Bone Pain after her chemotherapy treatments. Apparently, I had no clue what she meant. I've had issues with my back, neck, and knees and know what it feels like for the joints to ache or grind or hurt...Naively, I assumed my sister had aches like arthritis or a headache. Silly rabbit.

BONE PAIN DRAMATIZATION:

The Bone Pain (BP) gripped me in its clutches and twisted until it forced me to my knees. It started with a migraine headache: that spike behind your eyes and pressure that makes it impossible to open your eyes fully. Imagine that spike extending down your neck, spearing along your collarbones and shoulder blades before inexorably creeping down to your lower back.

With relentless intensity, the pressure grew. I tried shifting to different positions to avoid the pain in one area. A fleeting respite and then the pain resurfaced in a new locale. Repeat.

Can you tell I couldn't sleep Sunday? Sleep deprivation evokes my dramatic side. I threw a Vicodin at the BP, who chuckled at my paltry efforts. Feeling like I'd been drawn and quartered, I had to drag myself to teach Pilates yesterday morning. Luckily, my two clients are kind and forgiving and experienced. I canceled the rest of my classes.

After returning from Frogs, I took a Percocet AND an Ativan because I was feeling nauseous too. Take that Bone Pain! Finally, I slipped into a semi-coma for four hours; a brief respite from the unbearable pain.

Let's just say Monday was a waste. I did learn that Claritin is often given to help counteract the effects of the Neulasta BONE PAIN. I bought some yesterday, this is getting expensive, and I'm not sure if it helped too much. Next time, I know to take the Claritin pre-Neulasta shot. I'll also go to acupuncture for the Bone Pain too, since it worked so well for the nausea.

Note to self: do not get pompous about how well you are handling cancer treatment. I will be prepared for Round Two. Hopefully, no more surprises. Round Two comes with a wig.

This week I will focus on more friends, family, yoga, laughter and love to keep me floating on. And, I'm hoping to wake up in the morning sans the BP.

Thursday, March 18th: Humbled and embarrassed...

by the grocery shopping trip and the reasons behind it.
Spoiler to all my healthy, nutrition-savvy, holistic friends: I had no choice. I had to buy this stuff. Really. And, I've already started eating it.

So, I slinked into the grocery store incognito with sunglasses firmly in place. If one of my students saw me, it would be like the time I got caught red-handed at In-N-Out burger with a double-double at 10:30 am. Or at Wine Steals with syrah-stained lips and the remains of a four-cheese pizza. I had to be stealthy.

Yesterday, the nurse advised me to go for the bland, "d" diet. No fiber. No whole grains. Sodium to help with dehydration. Basically the opposite of healthy eating. I was actually going for sodium, which I avoid at all costs because I blow up like a puffer fish when I eat any salt. Soft, moist foods for my upset tummy.
My shopping cart: (copied from receipt for accuracy):
Jell-O Vanilla Pudding
Applesauce
Thomas' English Muffins (white)
2 Baking Potatoes
Tub of Shedd's Spread Mashed Potatoes
Can of Chicken with Rice soup (white rice)
Zantac

Bananas
Haagen-Dazs Low-fat Frozen Vanilla Yogurt
Ginger Snaps (ginger good for tummy)
Organic Low-fat Chocolate Milk (not recommended but,
I extrapolated)
Rold Gold Pretzels

There is a method to this madness. Let me explain.

This week has been challenging, to put it mildly. One minute I feel okay and then BOOM, something else hits me. Now, my bone pain seems better, just a moderate headache. I can handle that. I've also got some new preventative tips for the next go-round with the Neulasta shot. I cannot go through that type of pain again. Won't, shan't, can't.

Yesterday morning I taught my Pilates Group Reformer class and felt a step above okay. My stomach wasn't steady and I felt like I had a bout of stomach flu. Nonetheless, after teaching, I got on the reformer to attempt a mini-workout. Ten minutes and I was pooped. And, a little dizzy from being on my back. Humbling...

Next, I stopped to get some veggie juice and dropped into lululemon Carlsbad for a quick "hello." Within a matter of minutes, my energy level plummeted.

I returned home and promptly lay down for what appears to now be a habitual daily nap. My tummy continued to give me trouble. Can I be more euphemistic?

Did I forget to mention the little tidbit about buying a bottle of Mylanta on Tuesday night? And that I chugged it out of the bottle in the Vons parking lot? Do not put keys in ignition. Do not pass go. Do nothing before opening the bottle and gulping it down as fast as possible!

If I did mention it, it is worth repeating. Who am I these days? Is chugging Mylanta worse than chugging Mike's Hard Lemonade after the breast biopsy? Methinks yes.

After napping intermittently throughout the afternoon, I dragged myself up to teach my evening Pilates Group Reformer class. My stomach had other plans for me and I had to excuse myself a few times during class. Not embarrassing at all. Not one bit.

One of my students dropped off an amazing dinner for me at Frogs, and I promptly hightailed it home to share it with my friend Kirsten. It was absolutely delicious, but I don't think my stomach appreciated any invasion that was not a clear broth, ginger ale or absolutely white and fiberless.

Let's just say that my evening deteriorated to a point where I had a temperature of 99.7 degrees (100.5 means hospital), and absolutely no respite in sleep. At around midnight, I had to call and leave messages to have my morning yoga classes covered because there was no way I was getting out of bed, much less walking and talking. I just prayed that I wouldn't have to go to the hospital. I think I nodded off at 3 a.m.

After speaking to the nurses a few times, I was advised to go on an extremely bland, white-food, soft, fiber-FREE diet for a while. Potentially throughout treatment.

So, all of my virtuous pursuits into vegetables are on hold for a little while. Nothing that could upset the delicate organ that is my new stomach. The stomach that has been decimated by chemotherapy, pain meds, sleeping meds, steroids, anti-nausea meds, at least 10 different natural supplements and probably is just a gaping hole in my mid-section.

Time for dinner! Mashed potatoes, chocolate milk (organic) and some vanilla pudding for dessert.

Friday, March 19th: Breast cancer and yoga, things that make you go hmmmm...

I'm excited to be starting my Yoga for Cancer Therapy training at Prana Yoga Center in La Jolla tonight. I was reading my pre-assigned homework for this weekend's training and it gave rise to many questions that I would love answered.

An interesting article by Joanna Colwell called Re-Examining Breast Health suggests that yoga can help you optimize the health of your breasts. The frustrating thing is that all the experts agree that they cannot specifically tell you why you personally got breast cancer. Was it environmental factors? Genes? Lifestyle? Just being a woman who has breasts? That seems to be the one connecting factor.

The agreed upon primary factors:

You are a woman.
You have boobs.
Family History--Mother and/or sister.
Lifetime exposure to Estrogen: early onset of menstruation, number of pregnancies, breastfeeding.
Alcohol: one drink a day ups risk by 40% (how in the world did they come up with this number? Reported by people who get breast cancer? By people who kept a log for their entire adult lives of each and every drink? How accurate could this possibly be?)
High exposure to Radiation: chest X-rays, radioactive fallout
Stress: okay. Again, how measured?

It seems to me that most of these factors are out of our control. How old we were when "Are You There God? It's Me, Margaret" became a reality? Being born a female? Hmmm....it all seems so vague. And, while the experts can say things like a plant-based diet can help protect against cancer, they cannot say a woman got breast cancer because she was a vociferous carnivore. There is no clear profile of a breast cancer victim. Woman with breasts. That's it.

Before I get myself all worked up, I do agree that having a lifestyle where stress is minimized and healthy diet and exercise--including yoga--are emphasized, can be helpful in disease prevention. I can see it with heart disease, for example. I live that lifestyle.

Here are the questions I have and part of what I hope to learn in the connection between yoga and cancer in general.   How did I, who left the legal profession, then quit my high-stress corporate sales job to immerse myself in teaching yoga full-time, get breast cancer?

Was 20 years of birth control use a factor?

How can yoga help? I understand how it can help while going through treatment: reducing stress, boosting the immune system, stimulating the glands, encouraging lymphatic flow, calming the nervous system. But, how can it help before cancer hits? Does anything we do really prevent cancer? Can we ever know?

Did my car accident in December 2007 that culminated in an artificial cervical disc-replacement surgery in 2008 cause this cancer? Did the continual disruption of my yoga practice contribute? Maybe the X-rays and MRI of my neck caused breast cancer? Maybe taking out a disc and replacing it with a titanium and polymer one caused breast cancer? Maybe the stress of it all? Will I ever know?

I look forward to delving into this discussion. I also look forward to some nice meditation tonight.

Saturday, March 20th: New Moon is here!

I am finally feeling normal. I enjoyed half a cup of coffee this morning without any evil repercussions. No medications for two days straight. Well, except for the sleeping pill and that doesn't count. My body is finally not being hammered with chemicals. I can swallow my herbal supplements.

And, I don't need to subsist on potatoes. That aspect is bittersweet. It will be an every-third-week potato and ginger ale diet. Back to the vegetables and clean eating while my stomach can handle it.

The way I see it, I've got two weeks to work out and eat right to prepare for the second onslaught of chemo on April Fool's Day. Perhaps with this pattern, I can maintain. Cautiously optimistic.

The Yoga for Cancer Therapy training is wonderful. We've started both sessions with a restorative yoga class. I'm not accustomed to using bolsters and blocks and straps. This is a new area of yoga for me and I like it! I also think that I'll enjoy sharing it with others. My brain is a bit full, so tonight isn't the night that I will disseminate what I've learned. We've got another session tomorrow and another full weekend on April 2nd.

The course is bringing up a lot of emotions for me. When it was my turn to introduce myself to the others last night, I couldn't do it without tears. This morning, I woke up crying. I can't recall the last time I cried. The first month I

101

would wake up, climb in the shower, bawl my eyes out and then proceed with the day. Perhaps I am reaching a new stage in this process. Return to emotion?

Today is a good day. A few times, I almost forgot that I had cancer.

In fact, I had a long stretch this evening where it didn't cross my mind. *New Moon* was released today and I, of course, had to buy the three-disc Deluxe Edition. Overjoyed, I drove home from Target with my prize, changed into comfy sweats and parked myself on the couch to enjoy. No distractions.

All you *Twilight* doubters and haters stop! I love, love, love the books and movies and nothing you can say will change my mind. Anyone who has had a broken heart or an unrequited love gets it. Two hours of sheer bliss.

Time to put in Disc Two, with the six-part documentary and interviews with Muse. Or, should I put in Disc Three with deleted scenes and interview with the Volturi? Or, maybe I should save one for tomorrow.

Decisions, decisions.

Sunday, March 21st: Sunday

Cancer sucks.

Monday, March 22nd: Good enough to think

New Moon was excellent on the third viewing last night. Love it. Maybe I'll watch it again tonight.

The last few days have been interesting. Physically, I feel significantly better. I have a lot of energy in the morning and then around 2 p.m. I crash for a few hours. The new dilemma starts from not having such a huge focus on the physical body and dealing with my mental and emotional bodies.

Time to think.

Time to feel.

Stepping off the merry-go-round and realizing that I have cancer and will be in treatment for most of 2010. Yoga is all about living in the present and unifying the physical, mental and emotional selves. Simple concept yet not easy in practice. I was able to be present in my Yoga for Cancer workshop this weekend. When I exercise or am immersed in an activity, I can be fully present. Unfortunately, I cannot do yoga or Pilates or walk all my waking hours.

What I've discovered? It is not a challenge to slip into darkness. Yesterday was rough. My mind keeps circling back to the fact that I absolutely do not want to go through five more rounds, five more weeks of feeling terrible, and although I've committed to going through with it, the resistance continues to rise. I don't want to play anymore.

One thing I've been told repeatedly is that I'll know who my true friends are. I've discovered that I have more friends than I ever realized. It is very warming to my heart. Most people have been incredibly sensitive to the fact that I'm not going to be "Claire" all the time. They are empathetic with my limited abilities to interact. I've got zero ability to do more than keep it together on a day-to-day basis. I'll keep trying my best.

I am excited to be teaching again this week. I'll be teaching two weeks on/one week off for chemo and recovery. It will be a gift to be immersed in my passion again after a week off. Day by day.

Tuesday, March 23rd: A pretty good day

I'm so happy to be back teaching this week. It feels great to be around all the positive, healthy people! I am blessed to be able to teach others and focus exclusively on them for a while. And, it helps me keep the demons at bay. I feel the depression lapping at the edges constantly now.

Then I met Nancy, who is also going through treatment, at the lagoon for a walk. Batiquitos Lagoon is truly magical. It is comforting to be able to vent with someone who is going through the same unasked-for journey. To commiserate. To empathize fully. We both have energy in the morning and crash in the afternoon.

My dance card was full today. Next, I met Meredith for lunch at a new restaurant called Lotus Café. Meredith's lunch looked great, mine wasn't as tasty. Randi's vegetarian chili is the bomb and nothing could compare. I now know better than to order it anywhere else. It was lovely to catch up with Meredith. I think she may have promised to make me homemade mac-n-cheese. Pretty please?

As nap time now appears to be set for 2 p.m. each day, I made my way home. And, took a nap. Actually, these afternoon naps are more of a dozing fest. I'm not sure how much actual sleep I get, but the cats are very pleased with my new habit. Finally! Mama cat gets it. No napping alone in this house.

I taught this evening at 6:15 and again, it was fabulous to be in the studio teaching. Now, I'm ready for bed. At 9:15 p.m., Todd's already there. What's his excuse? It is his Birthday Eve and the sooner he sleeps, the sooner he is the official Birthday Boy.

No profound insights today. Just logging it in. One day at a time.

Thursday, March 25th: Shedding strands...

What a ride. The last few days have been intense.

The good: it was Todd's birthday yesterday. We went to lunch at Claire's on Cedros in the art district of Solana Beach. Claire's, besides having a lovely name, has excellent food and a charming, cottage-like ambiance. Later, we spent a quiet evening at home, toasting Todd's turning 41 with a Newton 2001 Cabernet Sauvignon that had been comfortably resting on its side for the last five years. My first taste of wine since chemo went down smoothly.

Teaching continues to go well. I am grateful to have such a positive world in which to immerse myself, if only on a limited schedule. Glimmers of panic pop up intermittently that I am not in a position to grow my business. In January, I was poised to expand my clientele, to maximize my new role as lululemon ambassador, to host a retreat, and to film some workouts for Exercise TV. And now? Holding pattern. Medical bills are rolling in and although my insurance is excellent, it doesn't cover everything. I am scared.

Physically, I continue to feel better each day. No nap today! I did sit by the pool for about an hour and my skin didn't react negatively to the sun, as the nurses cautioned me when I began chemo. Slathered in sunscreen, armed with *Twilight*: I finally found some solace. I'd realized that I'd read the other books in the series twice and had neglected to read the original more than once. *Quel horreur!* For some reason, I can just lose myself in this story. Anything that works.

I desperately need to escape. Why was I feeling so distraught last night and this morning? I've started shedding. When I comb my hair, several strands slip out in the comb. I'm talking four times the usual shedding that occurs. Mind you, I don't have a lot of hair. Seeing 20 at a time exiting at an alarming rate does not make for a positive attitude.

I know it is temporary. I know that this too shall pass. I'd even take that doctor slicing up my liver a few weeks ago again over this. Hair is important. Geez, I'm the girl who in high school had a terrible perm and haircut and literally wouldn't leave the house for two weeks. My hair is a comfort zone for me.

I'm not the ideal candidate for baldness or rocking the bald head. I see others do it. I know it can be done. I respect the women who can carry it off. I mean, I don't even wear hats, unless I'm in the sun. I've got a wig and will have the hat hair, but bottom line my bald head will be a constant visible reminder of cancer.

Regardless of which part of this journey triggered my despair, I felt hopeless this morning. It all feels like too much to bear: a battle with no true end in sight. I'm struggling with the contradiction of living day by day and consoling myself with these side-effects being only temporary. I feel like I'm missing out on living each day to the fullest. I feel caged. Restrained. Frustrated.

How to handle these up and downs?

I'm going to try more acupuncture for the depression/anxiety that I cannot seem to control. I'm going to remind myself of all the love and support that I'm blessed enough to have surrounding me. Nonetheless, with each passing day, I feel more isolated.

A friend suggested planning something fun in conjunction with each chemo round. Ever since I ran the animal rescue in LA, I've dreamed of visiting the Best Friends Animal Sanctuary in Utah. Todd and I began researching a trip in May, prior to Round Four. You get to volunteer with the animals all day and you can even take a dog for an "overnight" to stay with you while you are there. I am so excited at the prospect of going and just interacting with and helping the animals for a few days. Animals calm me.

I hope we go.

Friday, March 26th: Hair today, gone tomorrow

Yesterday, I left my hair in the Pippi braids all day. I was not equipped to resist hysteria and more traumatic shedding.

This morning, I had no choice but to wash the hair before I went to teach. Combing my hair, very gently mind you, resulted in it exiting in clumps. Whereas yesterday, about 20 strands would come out at a time, this morning it was more like 50. Once again, I was starring in a horror movie and couldn't escape. I clutched the hair in my hand, staring blindly at it before dropping it in the trash can.

In the shower, I cautiously shampooed and conditioned with a special brand especially formulated for cancer patients. As I opened the shower curtain, I happened to glance down and screamed at what appeared to be a tarantula crouched on my hip. The positive: it wasn't a poisonous spider. The negative: it was enough hair to convince me otherwise, if only for a second.

You'd think with all the shedding that I would have bald patches. No. My hair just looks really thin. With care, I slowly re-braided my hair. This hairstyle seemed to be the safest mode for preservation. I don't think I cried. I don't remember.

The speed of the molting convinced me that I couldn't wait until Sunday to buzz it off. It has to be tomorrow. I cannot endure two more days. And, who knows, I might have a bald spot by then. For some reason, more of the pretty blonde strands have exited and the grays are holding on tenaciously. It figures. The grays started showing up back when I was in law school and up until now, I've done a pretty darn good job of camouflaging them. Wow, no secrets anymore.

I taught my 10:35 a.m. Frogs class and it was fantastic. Love the yogis!! The room was saturated in beautiful, strong, calming energy. Thank you for providing this solace for me. I almost lost my composure a few times because when I'd bend over to demo a pose, my braids would shift with me. I was terrified one was going to just fall off and plop onto someone's mat. You know, like how in those zombie movies a limb would just drop?

I've summoned the troops to accompany me to Patti's house for the buzzing and wig fitting. Angie and Joanna are making the journey down from LA and some of the local girls are coming as well. I'm going to have to consume some liquid courage, most likely in the form of mimosas, prior to doing the actual deed. I just pray that I can handle this part of it with dignity. Doubt it.

Patti promises to custom fit my wig so that I can walk out the door with hair. I trust her implicitly. She is such an angel and as she is a survivor, she understands. My wig will look great and I'll feel fine. My hat hair will also be cute and I can mimic my Pippi braids with a baseball cap for working out.

Monday, I'm meeting with Lois, my acupuncturist and her mother, who does hypnotherapy. The original purpose was to give me some tools for handling this depression that won't stop knocking on my door, but I'm going to ask if she can suggest to me that bald is beautiful while I'm under.

It can't hurt.

Saturday, March 27th: Hair Removal: Part One

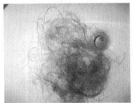

Today is the day.

When I showered this morning, the deluge began. I tried to catch some of the clumps and throw them in the trash can so they wouldn't clog the drain completely. What a milestone: my final shampoo and conditioner for around three months. No more highlights or haircuts. How much money will I save?

You, who have chosen to follow along my journey, cannot escape what I saw this morning. Sorry. This is the sink after combing my hair. Pretty powerful stuff. What is that old cliché? A picture is worth a thousand words?

I'll definitely be saving in waxing and shaving. Not to be too personal, but it is all part of the process. Being half-Mediterranean, I've always fantasized about not having any hair below my nose-line. And, I've spent a lot of money to remove said hair. My little sideburns pulled right out. My eyebrows and eyelashes seem unscathed for now. They better stay. Or else.

I do realize that this means the chemo drugs are killing the rapidly dividing cells. Is that the silver lining?

I went to the cat house at Petco this morning with my remaining hair carefully arranged into a little twist. And, I mean tiny. I'd lean forward and feel the clip shift slightly and was again afraid that the whole thing would just drop off and the cats would catch it like a toy.

The cats seem to sense my distress. Each one sniffed my eyelashes, brows and hairline and gave me a little kiss. They were all very sweet and mellow with me today.

Currently, I don't feel angry. I cannot pinpoint my emotional state. I am itching to rip the remaining mop off my head. The molting is, simply put, gross. My heart is racing a bit, perhaps my adrenaline is up, a thread of anticipation to just get this part completed.

I appreciate everyone's comments and confidence that I will look beautiful bald or with various head coverings. The jury is still out. We'll have to see après-shearing today.

I can confirm that with a scarf, I look like a 65-year-old peasant who should be leading a donkey, with water buckets over her shoulders. Trust me. And, for anyone who remembers my hair senior year at Oakton High School or in the spiral perm days of the late 1980s, you do know what a difference hair can make!! Bring on the buzzer. I'm ready.

Sunday, March 28th: Hair Removal: Part Two

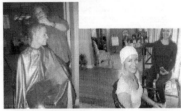

The Cat In the Hat on Claire's Hair
I have no hair
I do not care
My locks are gone
And I am free
I am beautiful bald
As you can see
Now in the mornings, my sweet dears
I do not brush
I do not fuss
So envy, envy, envy me
While you are primping, wasting time
I can change my look on a dime
I'm ready to go with a wig or a hat
Fast out the door
Now try and top that! (By Elizabeth Olson)

Mimosas are the best. Yesterday afternoon was a lot of fun. Really, I didn't even cry. Anne, Angie and Joanna and I shared mimosas and yummy snacks in preparation for heading down to Patti's for my shearing and hair fitting. Lots of laughter.

The mimosas went down so smoothly, in fact, that we realized we needed a designated driver to chauffeur us to Patti's. Enter my wonderful boyfriend Todd. Not only did he drive us down, he dog-sat Puffy, Angie's little dog, and picked us up afterward. Thanks Todd!

Patti made the experience fun despite a small snafu as my Pralines and Cream shade didn't come in on time. We've got to wait until April 6th. In lieu of it, we used the same wig style in a lighter blonde. So, I look like Cancer Barbie. The wig looks amazingly real. Patti custom fit it to my head, trimmed it to look more like mine. Really cool. I also absolutely love my hat hair. What fun to have long, thick blonde hair under my hats!! Let's just hope they don't blow off.

The shearing was interesting. Patti wisely positioned me away from the mirror. My remaining hair was so knotted that she just whacked it off. First, we saw what I looked like with a short, beveled bob and surprise, surprise: it was cute! Who knew? I guess since the last time I had a bob was when I had the bad perm in high school, I didn't think I'd ever look okay. I also like the "Posh" short wig and may get that too. Again, who knew?

When she brandished the clippers, I began to quiet. My head is very tender and the remaining hair feels very painful and sensitive to the touch. She had to stop because it was hurting me so much. I knew I should've brought a bottle of champagne with me!

Now, there are two main comparisons for my shorn head. A nun in a black-and-white 1960s French film or the women in the old Charlie's Angels episode where Cheryl Ladd was kidnapped by a maniac who kidnapped pretty women made them wear burlap robes and sheared off their hair. Either way you look at it, it isn't pretty. I'd like the remaining inch or so to be removed.

My head still hurts so I'm sitting here with nothing covering it. Hideous. But, I'm in the house and Todd and the cats are just stuck with it.

We're going for a walk later. I think it shall be the hat hair and baseball cap. HOT

Monday, March 29th: Baby steps...

Once the champagne wore off and reality set in, I realized I am bald. Bald, bald, bald. Although I was surprised to discover that my head is very nicely shaped. There was no way I was leaving the house. No walk.

To add insult to injury, I am not only bald, but my scalp is tender and painful. Patti recommended a baking soda and water poultice to soothe it. It wasn't pretty to have a white pasty cap, but it was magically refreshing and soothing. Putting the wig or even a hat on only added pressure to my already tender little head.

Rocking the baldness outside of the confines of the condo was not an option. Not happening yet. Or, possibly ever.

Today, I resolved to brave the elements. For Outing One, Pilates, I wore the wig. Unfortunately, I couldn't quite recall all the techniques to make it look realistic and natural so I resembled Miss Piggy. My students were kind, but I wasn't comfortable. I zoomed home and ripped it off and slapped on some baking soda paste.

For Outing Two, Todd and I walked at the lagoon. I sported the hat hair in a ponytail. It felt relatively natural. But, when I got home, my head was tender again. Back to bald. It just felt better to be unencumbered.

Outing Three was supposed to be teaching yoga. I chickened out today, however, and got a substitute. I just wasn't ready to face the world protected only with a thin cotton cover. I will do it tomorrow. I do like my cotton beanie and ordered three more in different colors.

I had some more acupuncture this afternoon to deal with the emotional rollercoaster that is my reality these days. I felt incredibly relaxed when I left. Then, I headed back to Patti's for a little wig adjustment. She showed me a few tips, like pulling out the little "baby hair" around my face to soften the hairline. That woman is a miracle worker. We'll see if I can replicate her handiwork when I try it again. I guess it will just take practice. It seems like a lot of work.

Enough about the hair.

How am I really feeling about this latest development? On one hand, I'm a little relieved because it is over. I am bald at last. The anticipation and the horror of losing my hair is over. It was one of the worst aspects of this journey thus far. Now, it is reality. No more anticipation. Just dealing with the present.

Round Two is my new reality. Dealing with the aftermath of Round Two will be my reality over the next week.

I cannot help but consider how this will impact my career. I thought that I was exactly where I wanted and needed to be. Perhaps not. There must be a reason why all my career plans are on hold. Why I cannot move forward. Why I can merely tread water by hanging on to some of my classes. I am clinging to the belief that the universe has something huge around the corner for me. Who knows what?

Over the last week or so, I've been reminded of my interest in life coaching. Originally, my idea had been to combine it with yoga to achieve a true balance between personal and professional life for my clients. Maybe this interim will give me the opportunity to delve into this concept more. An old friend, who is a successful coach, offered to work with me to explore the potential. Who knows?

My best friend Megan is coming out to stay with me for Round Two. She arrives tomorrow and I'm really excited to spend time with her, although it probably won't be that much fun for her. Selfishly, I'm thrilled to have her here anyway. The sooner I go to sleep, the sooner I get to see Meg.

Tuesday, March 30th: Trying to stay present

How to measure time these days?

The present: Megan arrived today and it is wonderful having her here. I taught three classes: one with hat hair and two in my little beanies.

Dramatic crisis this morning: the hat-hair elastic strap that goes across the forehead broke. I wasn't prepared to leave the house with only a beanie. So, I stapled it together and slapped it on my head to teach my *active.com* yoga class. Because the hat hair would melt in the heated yoga room at Sculpt Fusion, I braved it with the cotton beanie. I just avoid the mirror.

The future: Chemo Round Two is Thursday. I'm trying not to dwell on it, but I've got to start all the pre-treatments, aka steroids, tomorrow. Preparation for three hours in the lounge chair at Scripps. Preparation to get sick. Preparation for what is coming. I'm not dreading the actual treatment as much as the aftermath.

At least I don't have to worry about my hair falling out.

Chapter 4: April

Thursday, April 1st: Great News: Done with Chemo!

April Fool's Day! HA. Four rounds to go after today.

Round Two of chemotherapy: done. Like my first treatment, I went to Lois for acupuncture to help calm my steroid-amped brain. Steroids make me very talkative and intense. Imagine me in a good mood, magnified exponentially. Lois observed that the yoga class I taught this morning was incredibly challenging. Blame it on the drugs! Magician Lois relaxed me. I'm so lucky to have her help.

Megan came with me, which was really great. I love having her here.

I met with a different oncologist today, as mine is out of town. When we were discussing my bone pain, he called it "bony pain," which I found amusing. He tried to tell me that I should just use Tylenol or Advil for it. When I tried to elaborate how it had felt like being stretched out on the rack operated by a hooded demon during the Inquisition, complete with bones cracking and breaking, he stuck with his Advil guns. Um, not a job for Advil.

I had a different chemo nurse today, AJ. She was great. She gave me my Benadryl and Ativan along with more steroids, the T, the A and the C. Thus, I didn't have any reactions to the Taxotere this time. Yay. The only issue was that she placed the IV needle in a different spot, closer to my wrist. It was incredibly painful and remained so for most of the treatment.

117

Two girls who are going through treatment concurrently with me, Nancy and Lindsay, had their second round last week and told me that the side-effects were less intense this time. I'm optimistic that will be the case for me. Although, the chemo nurse told me that people like us who are young and healthy often have a harder time because we aren't used to being sick and rundown.

I'm predicting minimal bone pain and stomach upset this round.

I'm getting used to the bald head. It is actually very well shaped, almost good enough to go on a coin! I'm not ready to show it around in public and maybe never will. I'm alternating between the hat hair (shown in photo above), the hat to teach yoga, and the wig. The wig still feels weird, although everyone swears it looks natural. Day by day.

I'm really tired. She put some Ativan in the IV and I am a sleepy girl.

Round Two down. Four to go!

Saturday, April 3rd: Light at end of tunnel

What a great day at Yoga for Cancer Therapy teacher training! I cannot believe that the course is finished tomorrow and soon I'll be able to share what I've learned with others. It was incredibly nurturing to be surrounded by other yoga teachers, offering beautiful restorative yoga. Everyone in the class has such unique gifts and I feel like I absorbed some lasting lessons.

I did end up napping through the first hour after lunch, but the other students were kind enough to set me up on bolsters and let me snore. Namaste.

I felt better prepared for this round and am optimistic that I won't have such severe side effects days four through six like last time. I'm on the Claritin regime. I've got my best friend pampering me, cooking for us, generally being the Saint Megan that my father has raved about for almost, gulp, 30 years. Wow, 30 years. I'd say that is an enduring friendship. Granted, we met as toddlers. Oakton High School, class of...shhhh.

The steroids are wearing off and the headache behind my eyes is surfacing. I did attend training from 7-10 p.m. last night and 10-4 today, which is already intense without chemo involved. I do feel relief knowing that I've taken Monday and Tuesday off and there is no pressure to do anything but recuperate.

Let's see: more good news. Patti called me and my "permanent" wig is in. The wig I've sported this past week is very blonde. Can you say Pilates Barbie? The color that we've been waiting on, Pralines 'n Cream, is expected to arrive Monday and I should have it by Tuesday. It is much closer to the color that I lost last week and I will feel less conspicuous. To be honest, I love, love, love my hat hair. I feel like a cute, spunky little surfer girl. Now that I'm tucked in for the night, I'm sporting the bald head despite looking like an alien. A coin-worthy alien, that is.

Okay, the headache is kicking in. I've taken Tylenol every six hours, but I think it is time to keep ahead of the pain. Enter Percocet. I guess this entry will end soon...I will NOT experience the bone pain of last round again.

Emotionally, this is rough. I'm so blessed to have the support of my man, my friends, my family and my extended community.

But, last night was tough. I guess it is natural to cry myself to sleep and wake up crying. It has to be healthier to release the sadness and the pain instead of trying to bottle it up. The grace and radiance I am experiencing will outweigh the negatives. I know it. Back to my same theme of walking through the darkness and not pretending it isn't what it is.

The light is at the end of the tunnel. Everyone's love and prayers are driving me toward it.

Monday, April 5th: Fading Reflection

Somehow, I don't think I'll get used to that first look in the mirror in the morning. I feel like I'm disappearing slowly.

Inevitably. Like a painting fading in the sun, each time I encounter the reflection, it is fainter. My face, as I know it, seems to be eroding. The brows, the lashes, the color. Will I completely disappear?

Exiting the house is a process. I feel like an alien who puts on the mask, the fake hair and hat, the cloaks of looking "normal" prior to braving the rest of the world. As I sit here writing, I'm wearing my awesome cat hat and PJs. Catching glances of my bald head in the mirror over the last few days has been disturbing. I don't see me.

Compared to Round One, I'm doing significantly better. When the bone pain hit me last round, I was completely incapacitated. This time, I've been on Claritin and some meds in anticipation of bone pain and headaches and it seems to be helping enormously. I'm glad that I took off today and tomorrow to give myself the room and space to heal. My brain is floating. One minute, I feel completely present and almost normal and the next I am loopy. In fact, I would say loopy is an accurate current gauge.

This afternoon, Megan walked me and I ambitiously assumed a big jaunt. Fifteen minutes later, we re-entered the condo. Time is relative I suppose. Between Todd and Megan, I've been spoiled rotten over the last week. I wonder if Meg's husband Will would let us keep her? It isn't fair that he gets to have her all to himself. Lucky!

I completed my certification to teach Yoga for Cancer Survivors yesterday. In retrospect, I realize that it may not have been the most auspicious timing, but I did it! I hope to parlay all that I learned from the instructor and other participants to create a nurturing, healing class to help others. And, selfishly, it was healing for me to be in an environment like that as I battle this cancer.

Waves of chemo brain are rolling in and I'm feeling foggy. I'll sign off for tonight, but I am happy that this round seems to be milder and less painful. Knock on wood.

Tuesday, April 6th: No more Barbie

No panicked calls to the chemo nurses. No incapacitating pain. I can't believe that I feel so much better this round than last round. It is amazing.

Yoga tonight! Not wanting to think or teach, I just popped in the DVD and flowed with Rodney Yee for an hour. Part of the problem with this whole process, from surgery to testing to chemotherapy, is that I feel extremely disconnected with my body. My body has not felt like my own for three months now. Practicing yoga, no matter how gentle, reconnects my mind to my heart and body.

I'm glad that I took yesterday and today to recuperate and rest. Although I felt stronger today, I think it is better not to push it. Like I usually do. I'm still laughing at myself a bit for completing a full weekend teacher training the day after chemo...Rest is good. Rest is good. Rest is good.

I went to see Angel Patti today and swapped my Barbie wig for one that is more of a streaky, honey blonde. It feels so much better. Patti also thinned it out so I didn't feel too fluffy. When you've gone as long as I have with thin hair (the Spiral Perm Years notwithstanding), you cannot handle too much volume on top. I will try it out tomorrow morning.

I have spent more time on hair and makeup since I went bald than I usually log in over a year. Even just putting on the cap and hat hair is time consuming. I'll never take my flat little ponytail for granted again!

Today, I dropped Megan off at the airport. Todd is traveling for work. It is just me and the cats for 24 hours. The quiet feels right.

And, I've discovered another guilty pleasure: *Midnight Sun*. It is *Twilight* written from Edward's point of view. Everything makes so much sense from his point of view!! It wasn't published because someone leaked it before Stephenie Meyer was finished with it, but the draft is online. I'm trying to pace myself to extend the pleasure. I made myself practice yoga, eat dinner, and blog before I can return to it.

I'm so grateful that I have the attention span to read again.

Wednesday, April 7th: Just a quickie
Today started off fabulously and ended not so fabulously. Is that a word?

Teaching this morning was fun and afterwards, I completed a great workout on the reformer at the Pilates studio that left my legs feeling shaky. I've missed it.

It was a breathtakingly beautiful, sunny day in San Diego. I braved the pool for the first time. There was no way I was sporting faux hair, so I wore my big straw hat and pulled the brim down low and skulked to the far corner of the pool. I prayed that nobody would sit near me. A little reading and a little sunshine usually equals an hour of serenity for me.

Unfortunately, my day plummeted from there. My energy faded and my stomach started to ache. I don't feel like complaining, so I will keep it brief. By the time I finished teaching my 6 p.m. class, I was in tears. The wig pinched my head and gave me a splitting headache, but I didn't crack until it was over. Thank goodness for my supportive students. I love them! But, sometimes this is all just too much to bear.

Big silver linings of my day: first, we put in an ongoing search for the timeshare in Australia for September/October. Todd and I are finally going to Australia together and I cannot wait. Treatment will be complete, cancer will be gone, hair will be growing, and life will be good.

A more immediate event to look forward to: Best Friends Animal Sanctuary in Utah, May 6th through the 8th. Todd and I will stay in town; get a full tour of the sanctuary, and best of all, volunteer with the animals for a few days! Talk about miraculous therapy for the soul. Maybe I'll be cured after this trip and won't need any more chemo! I've dreamed of visiting and volunteering at Best Friends for years.

I learned about Best Friends back when I was Managing Director of Animal Avengers in Los Angeles. Best Friends is an animal sanctuary that shelters everything from horses and bunnies to donkeys to cats and dogs. When Michael Vick's diabolical dog fighting ring was discovered, Best Friends took 22 of the dogs: poor, exploited, innocent animals that had nowhere else to go. Best Friends provides a haven for abused, neglected and abandoned animals and also fights to protect animals nationwide. If you have never seen their site, visit www.bestfriends.org.

I feel better already.

Thursday, April 8th: A very good day

So many great things happened today. Hmm, I'm a lucky girl.

I just finished sharing dinner with my hot boyfriend. Neither of us could resist stuffing ourselves. Lori, the dinner fairy, cooked for us tonight and wow! This may have been the yummiest lasagna ever. As I sit here beached on the couch, I'm excited for another serving tomorrow. Oink.

Earlier today, my honorary little sister Melissa came to visit me. Melissa manages the Corepower Yoga in Pacific Beach and I haven't seen her since I put my classes on hold. We habitually had lunch after class most weeks, so we had three months to catch up on in one afternoon. Let's just say that neither of our jaws stilled for three hours. And, we didn't even get to discussing boys. It was fabulous! Sometimes you don't realize how much you miss someone until you see them again.

I taught my Sculpt Fusion and Active.com classes today. As usual, teaching made me happy. I love that I can teach, even on a limited schedule. After class, someone I'd never met before approached me and told me that they were following my blog and complimented me on it. How cool! This blog is incredibly therapeutic for me to write and it is gratifying to know that people care to read it.

Okay, I said I'd shut up about the hair, but I cannot resist. Although I am almost totally bald, for some unknown reason stubble remains, the opposite of male pattern baldness. It crouches atop my head like a dark, ugly crown. I can lightly tug it and it comes out in my hand. It is all over my pillow and inside my hats. But, this nasty shadow won't exit stage left. The blonde is gone, the light brown is gone, the silver is gone but this won't fall out. If I have to be bald, I want a Kojak-smooth head.

On that note, I'm heading upstairs to see if Todd can buzz the remaining offenders away.

Saturday, April 10th: Peeping out of the cave

I'm sticking my nose out of my cave, but not yet ready to exit.

The same black mood that hit me three weeks ago struck again. Not just dark, but hyper-emotional. I think I cried 10 times yesterday. I know that at this point after the chemotherapy, my blood cell counts are very low. Perhaps there is a correlation to my psychological state? All I know is that although my physical body is okay, mentally I am out of sync.

It all started five minutes before I was about to teach my Fabulous Frogs Friday yoga class. Fabulous because there is magic in that room! I can't pinpoint what it is, but it is a blessed escape for me and from students' feedback, they feel it too.

I digress. Imagine that. Back to my saga.

I ran into an old friend and co-worker that I've known for 13 years and haven't seen in two. We had been close and he was always a shoulder to lean on for me when I was facing challenges. A decade ago, those usually were misery at the job or turmoil from a melodramatic relationship. Mark would just patiently listen. I know he thought I was a train wreck and by all accounts, on any given day, I was. Naturally, I haven't seen him now that I am with the man of my dreams and love my work. Ironic?

Seeing him triggered me for some reason and I burst into tears. At the gym. Right before class. He was in the midst of telling me I looked great and I sobbed out "I have cancer and this isn't my hair" or some reasonable facsimile thereof. Of course, I couldn't have just said hi, let's catch up on the phone later as I'm going in to teach now. That would be too easy.

I was emotional at the beginning of class, but the yoga flowed in and my worries floated away. I had a surprise drop-in from the lululemon West Coast Community Relations gal Jessica, who was out visiting ambassadors. She gave me a new mat to product test. It is called The Mat or Le Tapis and it is big, it is hot pink and it is fabulous. I tried it out in my living room today and will bring it along with me to teach and practice. Love it!

Once I left Frogs, I went home feeling dark. If I were a big drinker, I'd have had a healthy dose of whiskey or a bucket of wine. Instead, Todd and I went for a walk at the lagoon. It helped to be outside in nature and beauty. Nonetheless, I was still snarky and unhappy when we got home as I had to take Oreo to the vet. My poor little guy hadn't been eating and was lethargic.

Oreo's health hasn't been quite right for the last year, and after five visits and $2,500, we still don't have a diagnosis. More blood work and tests. Over the last 12 months, he's lost two pounds. That may not sound like a lot, but it would be like you or me losing 50. His nickname used to be Fatty McPatty and now he looks like a bag of bones. Anyway, this, too, upset me greatly. Oreo got some IV fluids and seems a little perkier. The pathologist should have the results of the blood work on Monday.

Let's see, what else got me? It all started with a beautiful hat. The wonderful Shelley and her daughter Taylor knit me several new hats. Taylor makes hats for people going through chemotherapy. I love them. With my hat hair and cute hat, I feel like a blond Ali McGraw from Love Story. Oops. Didn't Ali McGraw die in that movie?

All day I was thinking of my mortality. For the majority of this journey, I've been staying positive. Silver lining, right? I keep believing that this is another challenge for me to overcome, another life lesson (not needed thank you very much), and a process with an end in sight. June 24th: chemotherapy done. August: radiation complete.

But, what if that spot on my liver is the spread of cancer? What if chemotherapy and radiation and all the holistic remedies I'm using just don't work and my ticket is up? What if I die? It is possible. I can't completely shy away from that line of thinking and deny that not everybody survives this disease.

To sink deeper into the abyss, I watched the episode of Sex and the City when Samantha had breast cancer. I'd never seen it and a few people had mentioned it to me. It might not have been the best day for me to watch it. Samantha losing her hair, getting chemo, trying on terrible wigs, saying she didn't want to look sick, that she didn't want people to look at her and not see strength...been there, felt that. I'm sure most women in my situation have. By 10 p.m., I knew I was burrowing into the house all weekend. No need to spread this mood around town.

This morning, I went to the cat house after the tedious process of securing the hat hair and painting my face. When I arrived home, I knew I was in for the duration. Luckily, I'm in the middle of a new book and have lots of workout DVDs and a new yoga mat. In the house, I am bald cancer girl and don't have to worry about trying to appear like nothing is wrong with me.

A nice long workout and yoga session relaxed me and I feel a tad closer to my sunny side. By tomorrow afternoon or Monday, I may be ready to face the world again. I will inch a little higher up this rollercoaster. Until then, no exit.

Sunday, April 11th: Genie in a bottle

As I predicted, today was significantly better than yesterday. I'm just going to have to ride these waves. A lovely friend left me a message that she visualized my cave as a beautiful place, with a Moroccan flair and satin pillows.

I'll elaborate on the cave visual: the I Dream of Jeannie bottle. As a child, I was obsessed with I Dream of Jeannie. Not only did I dress up as Jeannie for Halloween on more than one occasion, I also had a friend who had two genie costumes and we'd play dress up. More than having Jeannie's ability to blink and make wishes come true, more than rocking the pink outfit, I dreamed of running away into her magical, beautiful bottle. Voila. So, code word for going to the cave=I Dream of Jeannie.

Todd's been generously offering to get me a new pair of running/walking/hiking shoes for a long time. I have a big dorky white pair that I got on sale at Marshalls about two years ago. Not exactly top of the line in either function or fashion. Maybe Todd's embarrassed to hike with me and my giant white clodhoppers. Or, he's just generous.

In preparation to leave the house for the first time in what seemed like an eternity, I sported the wig. There is just something about the full wig, as opposed to the hat hair, that feels really weird and unnatural. Off to Road Runner Sports we went, along with half of San Diego County. If the sun fails to shine, San Diegans shop.

I found a very cool pair of Wave Rider Mizunos. Now I can cruise with the cool kids.

Next, we hit Home Depot. Now, I did promise Todd's mom that I wouldn't allow him to force me to go to Home Depot. Ever. It was my idea. We'd decided to spruce up our porch. We've got a great view and really cute patio chairs, but we'd killed off all the plants last summer.

We transformed the porch with a big Ginger Shell plant for the corner, two lavender flowering hanging plants, a tiny budding violet for a Santorini blue and white vase and finally, some bright yellow flowers. Notice I don't list the names. Despite being clueless on botany, I do have eyes and everything is gorgeous. Now, the porch is alive with life and color.

I did have to rip off the wig after this three-and-one-half-hour endeavor. My scalp is still tender and itchy. I definitely prefer the hats and hat hair.

After christening the shoes with a stroll, we practiced some yoga together in the living room. Todd made us a tasty dinner of Yellowfin tuna and asparagus. I'm feeling full and happy. Good company, exercise and shopping makes for a positive day.

Each time I teach yoga, I remind my students to stay in the present moment, to live in the now, to allow each experience to unfold naturally. I need to practice what I preach each and every day when I wake up. I accept the days like yesterday and Friday and welcome the days like today.

Or, maybe I can blink my eyes and wish it to be October, just like Jeannie.

Tuesday, April 13th: Really? I mean really?

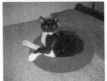

Yesterday was rough. Oreo, my 14- year-old cuddly love bug cat, was diagnosed with cancer. He only has months to live. I know they often say that pets mirror their guardians, but this is ridiculous.

I'm devastated. I adopted Oreo nine years ago from the Rescue House as a companion for my kitty Jake. Oreo is the cat that insists on sleeping curled up next to me, either in the crook of my arm or pressed up against me. He has given me immeasurable love and comfort over the years. I'm so grateful for him. I hate seeing him in pain.

He got a prednisone (steroid) shot today and we'll give him one once a month. It helps alleviate symptoms and will prolong his quality of life. Kind of like I get steroids with each round of chemotherapy to alleviate the side effects. I'll be spoiling him rotten. Well, spoil him more. I've always said I'd love to come back as a Petretti cat.

Since my natural defenses are low, this is trouncing me. Last night, I drowned my sorrow in the best vegetarian chili a la Randi, the entire pan of brownies she baked for Todd and me, and washed it down with a goblet of red wine. None of these pleasures could prevent me from bawling the entire evening. Chemo diet be damned. Losing an animal is so difficult because there are no negative associations, only pure love and affection.

Besides being focused on Oreo, I organized my medical bills and insurance. All I can say is thank goodness that I have kept my extremely expensive Cobra coverage from my former corporate job. A PPO, it covers a lot once my deductible is met. As I just discovered that treatment will end up costing around $250,000, yes, a quarter of a million dollars, I'm glad I had the option for that level of insurance coverage.

A sampling of charges:
One Round of chemotherapy: @ $9,000 plus
Neulasta shot day after chemo: $6,500
TOTAL: $15,000!!!

Most women endure four to eight rounds of chemotherapy. Plus surgery. Plus tests. Plus appointments. Plus a bucket of pharmaceuticals. We're talking roughly a quarter million dollars when all is said and done. How do people cope without insurance? Just give up and die? It is outrageous. Like we need additional stress. I'll bite back my healthcare tirade.

Finding the silver lining these last few days has been challenging. I did enjoy lunch with Lissa, who was the beneficiary of a big, fat emotional dump. Thanks Lissa: it means the world to have that kind of support. Friends and family are the light. Teaching was great tonight and another light in my life.

Back to the bottle. Genie bottle, not wine bottle.

Thursday, April 15th: Not loving the statistics...

What to write about today? How much I love my hot pink hat from Anita? Or, what has been weighing on me this week?

Back when this all began, I struggled a great deal with the idea of chemotherapy. In fact, I was convinced I would not do it. Until I was convinced that I should do it. Now, I'm circling back to my initial feelings that chemo isn't the answer for me.

Is that because of my bald head? The non-stop runny, bloody nose? The afternoon fatigue? The daily battle with not allowing myself to sink into depression? The frustration with feeling like my life is on hold until this treatment ends? Or perhaps it is the knowledge that I'm missing out on professional and personal opportunities left and right?

Initially, both oncologists that I consulted recommended six rounds of chemotherapy, with four being the minimum if I wasn't tolerating it well. Because I caught the cancer early and only had one positive lymph node, I really prayed to endure only four rounds. I am now obsessed with stopping after four.

Basically, my oncologist told me that if I can physically tolerate six sessions, I need to do it. Period.

But, I still just don't buy that chemotherapy is the cure-all. Again, I am feeling like this may be doing more harm than good. I'm concerned about the long term effects on my immune system. NO guarantees that it will work. In fact, my oncologist said that they just assume you are clear based on the statistics. What?

Then, I attempted one of my fruitless bargaining sessions with my oncologist. Good thing I don't practice law anymore because she wins every time.

I just read a shocking new statistic: survival rates from cancer have only improved five percent since 1950. Yes, only a five-percent improvement in the last 60 years. Contrast that with the cure/survival rates for heart disease improving 68% over the same time frame. And, recall, this treatment protocol I am on will cost $250,000 when all is said and done.

Basically, all the money and all the publicity and research have not improved chances of beating cancer in 60 years. How is that possible? I don't like those odds at all. Chemotherapy is a barbaric, poisonous stab in the dark. I will not receive a clean bill of health after two surgeries, months of chemotherapy and radiation. I will only receive an assumption that treatment worked based on statistics. And, I wonder why I feel like I'm going completely insane?

This week sucks. The sadness I feel about Oreo is weighing heavily on me. I'm trying really hard to focus on enjoying the present moment. Spending time with him. The positive parts of my day: the love, the friendships, the beautiful, enjoyable moments. We have eaten really well all week, thanks to Randi, Lori, and Christina's generous dinner deliveries. My energy level is just low, however, and I am miserable.

I bought a new book. Time to dive into some fiction and escape for a little while. Usually does the trick. Perhaps my sense of humor will show up on one of the pages. Let's hope so!

Friday, April 16th: Feeling better

I'm not bailing on the chemo regime. Hell, my hair is gone and I am invested in two rounds. I am just not happy about it. And, I'd really rather stop at four rounds instead of six. Perhaps if I say it enough, it will happen. Positive manifestation, right? Four, *quatre*, *quatro*, four, four, *four*.

Finally, today, I feel better. Some of the darkness has lifted from my brain and a little more light filtered in. Physically, I feel okay. Weird eye tics and bloody nose aside. I've had good workouts every day, including some restorative yoga this afternoon. I've eaten well and been consistent with my numerous supplements. I've received several calls, messages, cards as well as uplifting comments on this blog. It helps so much. I guess if there were ever a time I needed all the love, it is now.

The way my brain works is that something has to make sense to me before I can accept it. And, the lack of guarantees and grey areas of this treatment are challenging to reconcile. I wish I could have blind faith in treatment. Trust in the medical protocol would render this battle much more palatable. Acceptance isn't easy. I'm sure I will be kicking and screaming all the way to June 24th. Or, May 13th if my four wish comes true.

I don't have to BE anywhere or DO anything for the next few days and that feels fabulous. Some yoga, some long walks on the beach, some time with my kitties, some reading, some time for reflection. Ascending the road.

Sunday, April 18th: Sunrise

Hour by hour, day by day, my spirit is lightening. Not swift like a strike of lightening, but a gradual lifting of darkness similar to the sun rising on the horizon with shades of pink and purple streaking the sky. A dawning, if you will.

A walk on the beach, some yoga, a walk at the lagoon, some more yoga, some cuddle time with the cats. Time spent with Todd, time spent with friends both in person and over the phone, emails from friends, a special engraved spoon from Todd's mom. All contributions to lifting me up.

I received an amazing gift yesterday. A former co-worker, with whom I worked once upon a time in a faraway world called a law firm, heard about my cancer. His wife, a truly gifted artist, created the beautiful quilt pictured above for me. Patti even secured a tag on the quilt that says, "A Soft Quilt for a Strong Woman, Claire, we are thinking of you" from she and her husband Phil. The words on different squares are Energy, Humor, Love, Balance, Calm, Breathe, Namaste, Friends, Fearless and Hugs. Honestly, I am humbled and blessed by the grace of others throughout this ride.

Today, I had a conversation with Kim, one of my closest friends, who has known me for 19 years. When I was lamenting how I felt I was lost and in purgatory, she reminded me that I don't always have to be strong. Actually, her remark was more along the lines that she would be extremely worried that I was delusional if I did not feel depressed, freaked out, and concerned for my future. Thank you Kim, for always telling it like it is.

Part of my plan to remain afloat is to find a new yoga teacher or two that inspires me. I'm practicing at home, but would like to have a guide. I can't practice at Sculpt Fusion Yoga, the studio where I teach most of my classes, for now. The room is heated and it just doesn't feel good on my chemo-filled body. I need gentler yoga then what I am used to practicing and I feel like I'm starting over! So, I'll try some new studios closer to my house. I am convinced that my daily yoga practice is the tool to stay connected to my body and keep me present.

Finally, I'm not giving up hope that somehow I'll get away with four rounds instead of six. I'm generally good at manifesting what I want.

Here's a quote from Buddha focusing on the power of four.

"If you're respectful by habit,
constantly honoring the worthy,
FOUR things increase:
long life, beauty,
happiness, strength. ~Buddha~
Even if I end up with six, I still love this wisdom!

Monday, April 19th: A very good day

Today was a vast improvement. I felt alive and engaged.

Taught two Pilates group reformer classes and whipped my students into shape. It is so fun to create routines each week to challenge their bodies and engage their minds. I know they will all be thinking of me each time they walk up the stairs over the next 48 hours. Hee hee.

Enjoyed a yoga class at a studio where I've never practiced before with my friend Kirsten. It felt good to follow through on my goal to practice daily and reconnect with my body.

Taught my noon yoga class and felt inspired by my students' beautiful energy. Afterwards, I was able to catch up with my friend and fellow teacher Meredith at the always tasty Naked Café in Solana Beach.

Throughout all of it, I had energy. Positive energy. Fantastic. Savoring it while I can.

Now, it is time to gear up for Round Three on Thursday. Prescriptions to fill, blood to be drawn, appointments to make. Will this be the second-to-last treatment or the halfway point? Four, four, four: I can keep trying to manifest four, right?

I have my acupuncture appointments lined up. I'm convinced that the reason I haven't suffered any nausea with my chemotherapy is the skill of the talented Ms. Lois. Even conventional Western medicine recognizes the benefits of acupuncture in cancer treatment. All of the complementary therapies I'm doing help immensely.

If only acupuncture could help with the baldness.

Wednesday, April 21st: Round Three- Eve

I don't know why I feel the need to christen everything "Eve" as that generally denotes positive anticipation, but I can't help myself. Chemo Eve. Instead of Santa dropping down the chimney, TAC flowing through the IV. At least this round is the halfway point. Or, maybe the second to the last if you are with me on my Theory of Four. Round One seems distant in the rear-view.

My BFF Megan has returned for a second tour of duty in the chemo lounge. She is a brave soul. She brought me a present. It is a travel pack of shampoo and conditioner from L'Occitane for my fall trip to Australia. The irony.

Since my rough ride last week, I committed to rediscover my daily yoga, a.k.a. my sanity, again. Practice has been a challenge because the heat in the studios where I normally practice feels very depleting to my chemo-ridden body. Not an option. Most of the Frogs classes I enjoy are very intense and also not an option for the next few months. So, I'm now Yogini Explorer. And, I am experiencing an amazing week of opening.

I've sampled three new studios and enjoyed them all for different reasons. My mind-body-heart connection, which has been rudely disrupted since January, feels like it is merging back together. I feel lighter and softer. My right side, where I underwent two surgeries, continues to open up and heal. Yoga is truly magic.

And, I experienced a true *Celestine Prophecy* encounter this week. Remember that book? It was based upon the principle that there are no coincidences. In my yogic quest, I met Meredith Hooke, who owns a new studio called Asana Yoga Del Mar.

When our initial discussion began, we discovered that we both had grown up in Virginia. Cool.

Then: we are both from Fairfax. Small World.

Then: we both attended Pine Ridge Elementary School, Luther Jackson Middle School and Oakton High School. Really?!

Then: it got weird. During elementary school, she lived in Strathmeade Square. Strathmeade is a small development just a few blocks away from my childhood home. We each used to walk over to the nearby hospital to eat the French fries in the cafeteria. OHMYGOD!

Then: La Piece de Resistance: she moved out here because of her best friend. I knew said best friend from Pine Ridge Elementary School. I remember her because she was mean to me, probably because I had hairy legs, big buck teeth and braces when I was nine. But, I also ran into said best friend in San Diego 14 years ago because I replaced her as an associate attorney at the last law firm where I worked. Are you kidding me?

Um, I think there is a connection. There are no coincidences, right?

This week: exponentially better than last week.

Saturday, April 24th: Three down...

"To deny one's own experiences is to put a lie into the lips of one's life. It is no less than a denial of the soul." Oscar Wilde

I'm trying to recall the last few days. I feel like I've just emerged from a weeklong dream. Close! During the third round of chemotherapy on Thursday, I actually fell asleep. Or, passed out. Negligible details, right? I think the combination of Ativan and Benadryl with the TAC knocked me out. For days. I'm still fuzzy and piecing the last few days together.

I do recall that I taught yoga at Frogs yesterday morning, went by lululemon for a re-fueling of fresh spring tops. Passion and Lagoon: how can you not be fired up with colors like that? I'll be teaching the community class on Saturday morning May 1st at 9 a.m. Join me if you are local!

Let's see, that brings us to Friday afternoon. I received the infamous painful $6,500 Neulasta shot and acupuncture and Todd and I took Megan to the airport. We owe Will, her husband, for letting us borrow her for so long. There are no words.
I've been sleeping since then. Literally all day. My cats are very proud and have confirmed that I am, indeed, one of them. I dragged myself up out of bed a few times only to collapse back under the covers. I don't feel nauseous or ill, I just cannot keep my eyes open. Perhaps this is what people mean by fatigue increasing over time?

Todd runs the La Jolla Half Marathon first thing in the morning. This will be the third year that I greet him at the finish line. Meaning that I will drive down and meet him and not that I will be running the race with him. He always finishes in the top percentage for his age group and it is quite impressive.

I better go back to bed so I don't miss it!

Sunday, April 25th: Up close with the red devil

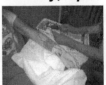

Apologies for the graphic view of the "A" drug but I love to share. This is the controversial drug where you are given a Popsicle because it dries out your mouth like the Mohave Desert. Also, the nurse must stay and administer the drug manually because if it spills it can burn your skin. Let's not dwell too closely on that information.

It is now Monday. I started writing this blog entry yesterday? Or, was it the day before? I feel like I've actually lost time. After the first two rounds, I did not sleep like this. I was up and about and one of the weekends even did the Yoga for Cancer Therapy training. What a difference a few weeks makes.

Finally, I'm deflating. Yesterday morning I bore a striking resemblance to Violet from the original Willy Wonka and the Chocolate Factory. Although my shade was pale pink not blue, my head and neck were swollen up like a big fat berry. Hideous. In fact, my eyes were so swollen that it was uncomfortable to keep them open. As a result, I spent most of the day resting.

Despite my repulsive condition, I was too stubborn not to drive to La Jolla to meet Todd. Probably not my brightest move as I couldn't see very well. Visualize the bulbous pink head, carefully camouflaged by sunglasses, hat and hat hair. The pressure from said accoutrements created terrible pressure and it is amazing my head didn't burst. Despite my efforts, I failed to find parking and didn't get to see him cross the finish line. He finished in the top seven percent again! Awesome!

Todd had a lot fueling him up and down those steep hills of La Jolla. In addition to his usual motivations, his maternal grandfather passed away on Saturday. His family is gathering in Warren, Pennsylvania, this week for the service. Todd leaves tomorrow. I wish that I were able to attend.

After a tough weekend, we were grateful to have a wonderful salmon and couscous dinner delivered, courtesy of yet another amazing Frogs yogini. I'm so grateful for the kindness and generosity of those around me. I cannot imagine this journey without it.

Tuesday, April 27th: The Incubator

Thanks to some rest with the cats, some good friends and lots of love in the air, I am gradually coming back to life. I still feel weak, tired and not particularly peppy, but it is only Tuesday night, right?

Over the last few months, I've wrestled with the paradox of "this is only temporary" and "live in the present." Certain things lend themselves to the realm of temporary, like puffy eyes, upset tummies or extreme fatigue. I know that I won't resemble Uncle Fester forever. I will eat cruciferous vegetables again without fear. And, my "Claire-level" energy will return.

Certain things, however, do not lend themselves so well to this premise. This is my life, dammit, and I want to live every minute of it. For me to be fully present, I need to experience, I need to live, and I need to be involved.

Sight, sound, taste, smell, feel. Passion. Intensity. 100%. Sacrificing to the halfway, the mediocre: not for me.

I'm not saying that I don't need my quiet time. Yoga, meditation, lazy naps with my cats curled up around me like two sleek guardians. I love to lie on the couch immersed in a good book. I enjoy lounging in the sunshine with a frivolous magazine. Not because I have to. I don't do well with being told what I can or cannot do. Cancer treatment is no different.

My day was highlighted by two wonderful conversations with two very different women, both of whom I have not seen in far too long. Both beautiful, wise blondes that I met at two really lousy jobs in Los Angeles that yielded really cool friendships. Maybe I've had so many jobs because I needed to find all these amazing friends that grace my life now? Thank you Jenny and Camille for the wisdom, love, and comfort.

The sage Camille offered some concrete nuggets for me. To help my existential struggle with the same old questions, she suggested a reminder of "this is why I decided to do chemotherapy." Back in February, I decided to have chemotherapy based upon all the knowledge and input I had gathered at the time. Tap back into the reasons I said yes to the drugs. I shouldn't second guess myself now.

And, Camille created the Incubator concept. She suggested that instead of being "on hold" or "treading water" during these months, perhaps I'm just incubating. A higher level of brilliance is percolating, something that I'd dared not even dream to date. I need to be a bald, little egg while this transformation occurs and I can then blossom into my full potential.

143

I like it. For now, I'll continue covering my bald little head with warm hats and fake hair, knowing that I'll emerge somehow new come summer.

Thursday, April 29th: Shifts

Another beautiful day in San Diego. I'm happy that I was able to get outside and enjoy some of the sunshine.

Today I walked for 30 whole minutes! Thirty minutes may not seem like a lot, but yesterday my legs were wobbly after a mere 16. This was no power walk. An old lady with a walker, an ancient three-legged dog, and just about everyone else on Paseo del Norte passed me but hey, I was disguised in my wig, hat and dark glasses.

Lots of shifts occurring this week that I didn't envision even a month ago. I realized, after being walloped by fatigue this past week that I need to conserve my energy to heal. Perhaps this has been obvious to everyone else, but I felt good enough to teach all my classes before. Now, I'm tired. I need more time to rest, reenergize, and recuperate. Yes, I put that in writing: Claire needs to rest more. What the heck will I be writing a month from now?

So, I made a tough decision to put my on-site yoga classes at *Active.com* on hold until I'm finished with chemotherapy. I've had to cancel so often, making it too erratic. We will re-launch the yoga program in July. I've also put another class at Sculpt Fusion on hold until the end of treatment because the heat is just overwhelming. I will return!

This week has been marked by discussions with a few clients and new acquaintances who were seeking advice because their doctors had severely restricted their exercise regimes. I, too, had these issues after cervical disc replacement 18 months ago and the two breast cancer surgeries in February. I'm still limited from the recent surgeries and chemotherapy. A 16-minute walk and some yoga was all I had yesterday, but it made me feel better.

Discussing these types of limitations is sparking an idea for writing an article to help others maintain activity and sanity while they recover from injuries or illness. I'd love to use my teaching and personal experience. I'm going to retreat to my I Dream of Jeannie Bottle-Incubator to percolate.

Friday, April 30th: TGIF

I'm so glad it is Friday. A protracted wobbly-legged week is over. Next week at this moment, Todd and I will have completed our first stint volunteering at Best Friends Animal Sanctuary. I can't wait.

We went for a walk at the lagoon and although the pace was painfully slow and I had to sit on a bench for a small rest, it was lovely. I know that each day I'll feel stronger. I'm motivated to feel strong next week to volunteer with the cats and dogs and visit Zion National Park.
My mind has been a rollercoaster of shadow and light, possibilities and dreams, pondering and percolating. Incubating mode.

I need to get a good night's rest before teaching at lululemon tomorrow morning. Can't wait!

Chapter 5: May

Saturday, May 1st: A Perfect Saturday

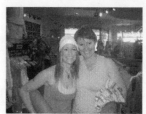

What a fantastic morning!

Fifty-four people attended the free community class I taught at lululemon Carlsbad this morning. Many of my regular students from Pilates, the yoga studios where I teach, *active.com*, and daily life came in to support me. Thank you for making it a very special morning. We packed a lot of fun into a small space. I love teaching.

I'm still riding high on the class this morning. I'm not sure if people realize how uplifting it is to see their smiling faces. When I'm teaching, I'm in a zone where nothing else matters except for providing a beautiful practice for my students. My goal is for my students to be fully present on the mat and to enjoy themselves. And, the gift for me is that I am fully, truly present.

One of my favorite people on earth, Jessie, attended. I got to meet Jessie and Justin's new baby: the perfect Justin Daniel Junior. Adorable! After class, I took Jessie into the bathroom to see my bald head. She astutely observed that it must be a lot of work to don the hair, the hat, the makeup before leaving the house. Exactly. Oh well, at least I can leave the house, right?

Because my physical strength seems to be returning, I'll embark on a longer walk today. Todd and I are going down to the ocean to enjoy the sea breeze and sunshine. We are so lucky to live within a mile of the beach! Later, I'm surprising Todd with a nice, romantic dinner out. I'll create a smoky eye; wear Sheila on my head and stilettos on my feet. I will feel feminine and sexy again if it kills me. Or, if it takes a few hours of preparations.

Time to bask in a perfect Saturday afternoon. No worries. Cancer doesn't get to hold court today.

Sunday, May 2nd: Beat the Second Sunday Curse

The dreaded second Sunday after chemotherapy. The prior two Sundays were woe-filled dark days where nothing could pull me out of my chemo-induced depression. Could the curse be beat?

I am happy to report that the answer is Yes!

I continued to ride the Saturday morning high into the evening. Todd and I had a romantic dinner at Firefly. I tamed Sheila and wore her with authority. It still feels weird to wear a wig and I cannot wait to have my own hair again. Nonetheless, we had a great night and went to bed happy.

I started the morning with yoga followed by a little nap with Jake and Oreo. My energy level is definitely still low. I hope it returns. I can't keep chugging vegetable juice hoping for a Popeye moment! My legs still resemble a newborn deer. Tomorrow they will be stronger.

Four sleeps until we leave for Best Friends!

Monday, May 3rd: Courage and Fear

May is working for me. Third excellent day in a row. Let's maintain this ascent.

A few recurring themes continue to arise. Fear and courage. Bravery and weakness. My friend Colleen sent me a handmade prayer shawl, filled with pure positive energy. Accompanying the shawl was a copy of a sermon on fear. It resonated.

Throughout this process, people are constantly praising me for my bravery and strength. I don't feel brave. Or, particularly strong.

Courage? Half the time I feel like the Cowardly Lion shrinking away from what comes next. I cannot bear the thought of three more rounds of chemotherapy. Or, shall I say, the cumulative side-effects of three more rounds of chemotherapy. I. Just. Don't. Want. To. Go. Again.

But seriously, I don't think that I am handling this in any more courageous way than others dealt a similar hand. For example, my sister Yael went through breast cancer five years ago and powered through it with the fearless grace she always emanates. She didn't seem to worry about some of the issues tugging at me, like the hair. She just did what she had to do.

When I say I don't understand why people tell me I am brave, I mean it. I don't know how else to handle this. I am just doing what I have to do to get to the other side.

Am I afraid? Fear is an interesting concept. After losing three brothers and one dear friend, perhaps I feel like I've faced death already. I truly don't fear it. In fact, I haven't considered it an option. I'm too stubborn to not morph into an old bat. I've got plans of careening down Highway 101 in a big Cadillac, you know, the 90-year-old raisin that can barely see over the steering wheel? Yelling at all the other drivers to clear the way? Not so different from today.

I'm not afraid to make a fool of myself. I'm not afraid to push boundaries and try something at least once. I've been called reckless and I've been accused of being an idealistic romantic. I've made many mistakes, some of gargantuan proportions. Yet, I really don't regret any of the less than stellar judgment calls. Because I was fearless. I was living life in the way I knew how.

What do I fear now? That life will pass me by as I'm in my incubator bottle. That I will miss out on important events in my friends and families' lives because I'm so focused on this battle. That I won't be there for those who need my support.

Fear: it won't rule my life. It cannot. Like Marianne Williamson says, everything in life stems from either love or fear. Everything.

I choose love this time around.

Wednesday, May 5th: Down dog in six weeks
May continues to be significantly better than April.

When I first began writing about the silver lining in this journey, I wasn't sure where it would appear. Thus far, it has shown itself primarily through my interactions with others. Some are people that I didn't know very well who have shown me how generous and kind they are. Some are my friends and family who have reminded me why I'm blessed to have them in my life. Some are people that I would never have met but for the breast cancer.

Today I spoke with an amazingly brave young woman, Kristin, who at age 28 learned that she had the breast cancer gene. She discovered this because her cousin was diagnosed at age 39 with Stage IV breast cancer and passed within a year. The standard protocol with the breast cancer gene is to have a prophylactic double mastectomy and also have the ovaries removed. Kristin had the double-M and reconstruction. Oh yeah, she'd just gotten married. 28 years old. How can this be right?

Almost every day someone tells me of a friend or colleague who was just diagnosed. The diagnosis of breast cancer in young women is reaching epic proportions. Why is this happening? In the 1970s the statistic was one in 20 women; today it is one in seven. And, the age of diagnosis continues to be earlier and earlier.

Kristin and I commiserated about how hard it is to be sidelined by all of this. We both are used to being very active and physical. Neither of us will accept that we can't get back to our regular routines. Despite what some well-meaning folks in the medical profession advise. For example, I was told by a physical therapist specializing in lymphedema that I shouldn't even try to do a Downward Dog for six months. Ha! It only took six weeks. (This photo was pre-surgery nonetheless)

The cancer can have some of my time. Not all of my time.

And, I'm leaving it behind while Todd and I head to Best Friends in Utah this weekend.

Saturday, May 8th: Milestones and Best Friends

A quick entry from Best Friends in Kanab, Utah. I think this photo says it all. This is Bari, a Catahoula Leopard Dog or a Catahoula Hog Dog. Reputed to herd cats. She and her brother were two of the sweetest puppies I've ever met. Good thing that Todd and I didn't drive here or Bari would be herding Jake and Oreo.

Please note that I am not wearing Sheila or any of my hat hair. Just the hat. A milestone for me. Building upon a milestone for me from Thursday morning when I taught my Sculpt Fusion Yoga class bald. No hat. Bald. Bald. Bald. I did wear Sheila on the plane and probably will wear her home too. Easier. Enough about the hair for now.

Nothing could have prepared us for the breadth and beauty of this sanctuary. We had a tour yesterday morning, which encompassed over 3,800 acres containing cats, dogs, horses, pigs, goats, birds, bunnies...heaven.

We volunteered yesterday afternoon and all day today. We walked lots of dogs, took Sasha for an outing to Angel's Landing, Todd took April for an outing this afternoon while I played in the Casa del Calmar, one of the Cat World buildings. Let's just say we have both been experiencing pure happiness and peace of mind.

So many people here are on return visits. It is just so cool to be around all these animal lovers who come here to spend time with the homeless pets. Todd and I definitely will return as this is the perfect annual trek. I've been doing rescue work for about 15 years now and I've never seen anything like this. Love, love, love it!

This trip has been on the "list" for five years. Check!

Monday, May 10th: Caught in public naked...

cancer style.

Yesterday we went to Zion National Park and hiked in the striking beauty of the red rock cliffs. The sky was a brilliant blue, the sun was shining and emerald-green trees and water surrounded us. We were in full vacation mode after two fantastic days at Best Friends.

And, then, my worst nightmare since I've been bald occurred.

The disaster occurred as we were descending the trail from the Upper Emerald Pool and moved aside to allow some hikers to pass us. As I stepped out of the way, a tree branch caught on my cute cream hat and yanked it off. Exposing my bald head. I felt naked. Vulnerable. Hideously ugly. Like the only person in the world with cancer. I cried. And, I couldn't recover for the rest of the day.

Since I began wearing Sheila and hats with hat hair, my biggest fear has been that someone will pull off my hat, revealing my bald head. For example, when we were at the movies, I was convinced that the person behind me was going to ask me to remove my hat. I didn't wear the hat hair to fly to Utah because I was scared that the security officers would make me take it off for some reason. Fear, fear, fear.

I hate being scared. Nervous. It just isn't my personality.

Perhaps the baldness represents everything that I hate about this journey. Just like my breasts are part of my identity and my femininity, so is my hair.

152

And, I just don't want people that I don't know to look at me and immediately be privy my biggest life battle. Can't I have my privacy? That may sound hypocritical since I am blogging for all to see, but it is different for me to sit here in the privacy of my home writing on the computer.

Standing bald on a trail in Zion, with healthy people surrounding me rendered me helpless, isolated, and utterly alone. Solitary on my journey. I couldn't shake that feeling.

Whereas at Best Friends I felt "normal" in just the hat, it didn't feel that way at Zion or in the airport or the airplane on the way home. The stewardess was just a little too cheery; the security officer who checked my license was too kindly. It felt like pity.

Overall, the weekend was incredible. I cannot stop thinking about all the animals that we encountered. Best Friends will definitely be an annual trip. We loved it. Happy times.

Three days to Round Four.

Tuesday, May 11ᵗʰ: Keeping it together...

I started reading an interesting book called *Close to the Bone, Life-Threatening Illness as a Soul Journey,* by Jean Shinoda Bolen. My sister shared it with me because it helped her cope with her own experience with breast cancer five years ago. Bolen employs several myths to illustrate how cancer affects us. In particular, she discusses the myth of Persephone from Greek mythology:

...a biopsy reveals cancer, through whatever means we learn of a life-threatening illness, the effect is the same: Persephone--the assumption of youth and health, the assumption of safety and immunity from disease and

death--has been violated and taken into the underworld......Illness as a descent of the soul into the underworld is a metaphor that brings to the intuitive mind and knowing heart a depth of understanding that cannot be grasped consciously otherwise...p. 15, Close to the Bone.

I've only begun the book, but her premise that the body cannot be separated from the soul resonates deeply.

Today is one of those days where I am doing everything in my power to maintain a positive attitude and still feel off. Why won't my darned brain comply with my wishes? Why are my mind and body not syncing?

I love lists. I love checking things off lists. Here goes: Things I did on Tuesday to feel better:

Taught yoga at Frogs. Check.
Walk at lagoon, listening to Guns n' Roses. Check.
Practiced yoga at home. Check.
Cuddled with the cats. Check.
Touched base with friends. Check.

Why don't I feel better? I feel tired and melancholy. My body does not feel like my own right now. It is bloated and puffy, as if somebody inflated me with a bicycle pump. No fair: if I am bald, I at least get to be skinny, right?

Onto the positive column: I am picking up one of my oldest and dearest friends from the airport tonight after I teach my 6:30 p.m. yoga class. Kim is coming in from Atlanta to be my sidekick through Round Four. We've had a wide variety of experiences together, like when we were in Marbella and Paris in 2001 or in Barbados for law school-summer school in 1991, or tubing down the Chattahoochee River with the Morins in Atlanta in 1997 or was that 1998?

I am so grateful that she is coming out to experience one of the less fun times with me. Just as Megan was a pillar of support for me during Rounds Two and Three, Kim will be too. And, I'm glad to give Todd and all my "local" friends a little breather in this seemingly never-ending saga. Despite my best efforts, I am dreading this next round of chemotherapy.

Joy, joy, happy, happy. Repeat 100 times...

Thursday, May 13th: Chemo-Eve Round Four

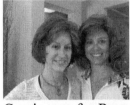

Gearing up for Round Four this afternoon. Kim and I will head to Lois' for my acupuncture and then down to the Chemo Lounge. After today, I'll only have two rounds left. More than halfway to the finish line. Hallelujah!

We had an awesome, busy day yesterday. Pilates, manicure/pedicure, lunch at the always yummy Swamis Café. It was gorgeous outside, sunny and 68 or so. Perfect. Then, we did the not-so-fun tasks of taking me to Scripps for my blood work. It doesn't become any more pleasant with repetition. After that, onto the magical Patti's house for some more wig tweaking and the selection of the new short Posh do. We had a blast trying on some silly wigs while Patti styled and trimmed Sheila. Now, Sheila is perfect!

Big news...drum roll...I'm going for the auburn Posh. Why not? Maybe I'm finally going to have fun with this. Sultry redhead one day, sexy blond the next and bald egg in between.

Last night, I had my dear old friend Kim (met circa 1991) and my "new" friends meet up at Third Corner. That place is so fabulous. Lissa, Kirsten, Meredith and Anne all showed up to eat, drink and toast off this round. I'm so blessed to have such beautiful, generous, smart, funny, kind friends. Lucky, lucky, lucky. Thank you all!

I've decided to have a big party at the end of chemo. After June 24th. I'd like to take a page from my friend April's birthday party last fall and make it a wig party. Everyone must wear a wig to be admitted and consume tasty cocktails. April's party was so much fun: talk about an icebreaker or two? Purple mullets, pink bobs, Bob Marley dreads...it will be a blast!! Start planning now...we'll have prizes!

I'm trying not to stress over how this weekend will unfold. I hope that I'm not as fatigued as I was last time, but as my legs have been feeling really tired, I have a feeling I may be on my back a lot. Sigh.

Friday, May 14th: Round Four: So far so good

I cannot stop laughing at the photo of Kim and me in those silly wigs. Trust me; you won't see me sporting either of them. I guess there is a style for everyone, right?

I much prefer my real hair circa February 2nd, 2010. How long will it be before I'll have hair that length again? Sigh...

Round Four went smoothly. I lounged on a bed because the recliner chairs were all occupied. It was fine as my legs were tired and this way they were elevated the entire time. Afterwards, Kim and I went and got mystic tans. God forbid she return from California pale! It was interesting to use the booth without having to utilize the shower cap. Is that what bald men do?

Today was a steroid-fueled whirlwind. Kim took her third class of the week with me, this one at Frogs. Then, we hit lululemon. Next, lunch at St. Tropez, then more shopping. Scored three pairs of awesome sandals at Marshalls. Four-inch wedges for Chemo Round Five.

Aftermath: collapsed on the couch. Whew. When will these steroids wear off? Maybe I'll be getting off easy this round! Or, perhaps because my Neulasta shot was delayed until Monday I'm not getting side-effects from that yet? I'll just hope for the best.

Kim and I had an awesome visit. It really didn't feel like I was a cancer patient at all! We had too much fun with all the visiting, sunshine, eating and catching up. I'm so grateful for my friends and family. Thank you, thank you, and thank you!

Saturday, May 15th: Incubation weekend

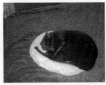

It is 8:12 p.m. on Sunday night and I only recently got up. The. Entire. Day. Was. Spent. Sleeping.

If indeed this journey through cancer is a time for me to cocoon and rest while brilliance percolates, I made a great deal of progress today.

My eyes are getting heavy...back to work.

Monday, May 17th: Nuggets from January

So, Round Four Incubation Period. I just feel like a giant sloth, slinking from couch to bed, bed to couch. If something is percolating, it is buried deep. In an effort to do something, anything, for the first time in days, I cleaned out my nightstand drawer.

Cleaning out the drawer did indeed trigger movement. I keep a lot of my random writing in the drawer. Four separate notebooks, as a matter of fact. Musings, partially written stories, ideas, and journal entries. Each time I re-read some of my ramblings, I get stimulated to ramble some more.

I discovered the notebook where I was scribbling the few days prior to and after finding the lump. It is surreal to look back and realize what an enormous turning point the second of January was; a day where I was full of resolutions and determinations for 2010. This was definitely going to be my year. On the 1st, Kirsten and I went for a walk on the beach and enjoyed a spectacular sunset, full of innocent dreams for a really big year. Not this kind of big...

Looking back at the past revealed something that got lost in the madness of these last months.

On January 2nd, lump day, Todd and I went to see 'Up in the Air.' We enjoyed the movie, but what stood out for me was that Sam Elliot had a small part in the movie. The actor always reminds me of my late brother Paul.

It sounds crazy, but every time I see a movie featuring Sam Elliot, I feel that my brother Paul is reaching out to me. I generally cry each time. When Sam Elliot stares out of the silver screen, crinkling his eyes and smiling slightly over his horseshoe moustache, I always feel a chill down my spine. Until I re-read my journal entry, I'd forgotten that Paul had played a part of discovery day.

Moreover, it appears that I knew immediately that the lump wasn't just a bump. Reading those words from a mere four months ago is striking. I also re-read a letter from Megan, after she'd read my blog entry about the drain. I certainly hated that damn drain, didn't I? It was the center of my universe for 12 days and, I must say, it still ranks up there as one of the most unpleasant parts of this ordeal. I still wish we could've made it a piñata. It feels like a lifetime ago.

I wonder how I'll feel in September, re-reading this blog post. What new insights will I find? Where will I be physically? Emotionally? Mentally?

Wednesday, May 19th: Always look on the bright side of life...la la...la la...la la...la la

I haven't felt like writing because I've been feeling so abysmal that I didn't really want to release that energy out into the universe. God forbid anyone ever read my private journal where I really vent! I'm swimming up from rock bottom so, here goes.

As I discussed last time, I cannot believe that four months have elapsed and that I am in the midst of chemotherapy, baldness, weakness and cancer. The cycles of treatment really do vary, although they are apparently the same. The fatigue is depleting my muscles. My legs are two lead bricks. What is a lead brick? The heaviest thing I can envision at present.

Anyway, all of my limbs feel like I am wading through molasses. Although I'd really like to go for a walk, I just cannot. Yesterday, we went for 15 minutes and Todd half pushed/half carried me up the hill into the door.

I meandered around Target for a while today, earning my spot in the Facebook group, "I went to Target for shampoo and spent $150."

Well, my title should be I went to Target for anything BUT shampoo, right? Nonetheless, I worked the aisles, and rewarded myself with a new lip-gloss, and not one, but two books that look interesting enough to finish. I barely restrained myself from purchasing the lovely blue Team Edward T-shirt. I want it. If someone happens to buy it for me, in size Small, I will wear it. In public. Hint. Hint. (Team Edward. Size Small)

I choose to count the Target excursion as 30 minutes of exercise. Anything not flat out on my back, as I currently am, counts as activity.

Tomorrow will be an intensive rest day, complemented with an afternoon massage. Maybe a good deep tissue massage will stimulate these semi-worthless limbs. Another strange side effect that is impacting me for the first time is some tingling and numbness in both my feet and hands. I can't recall which of the three drugs, T, A, or C causes it but I feel it. While I stand or walk. Currently, my left wrist is tingling. I am officially a science project.

Needless to say, I am crabby and not particularly friendly today. Poor Todd, having to live in the cross-fire. I am sorry, my love.

Today, I personify my pet peeve person. You know the one who wants to just dump all their problems in your lap but doesn't want to lift a finger to try to solve them? The emotional vampire? Yes, that is me. I have a tough time abiding the victim mentality, but it looks like I'm wallowing in it. No suggestions, no silver lining, no bright side of life. (Insert Monty Python "Bright Side of Life" song here)

I can confess all my darkness because I am rising above it. I can feel it. Soon. And, my favorite person, Randi, did drop off her super-sinful, perfect, delicious brownies.

There isn't much that a tasty, homemade brownie cannot fix.

Thursday, May 20th: A little clarity

Today, Doomsday is ebbing away in the horizon. Today, I walked on the beach with Todd and enjoyed the soft air washing over me as the waves broke on Ponto Beach. Today, the effects of Round Four are fading. And, today, I finally felt clarity and certainty about my career direction.

My cleaning out the nightstand drawer was just the beginning. I spent several hours organizing my beautiful file cabinet. New file folders, new labels with varied color magic markers, a place for everything, everything in its place. I cannot tell you how happy this makes me. I've now got my Yoga, Pilates, Fitness, Writing, Coaching, Goal Setting, Cat Rescue, and of course my Personal files all set up properly. I pared down and am now primed to move ahead.

Yes, I am a colossal dork.

But, I feel fantastic and ready to take the steps that can implement all I want to do. Whereas I've been feeling suspended since January, I now feel free for forward progress. It feels fantastic.

This cancer can have part of my time; this cancer cannot have all of my time.

Friday, May 21st: Rolling, rolling, rolling...

This fourth round aftershock is really a rollercoaster. I thought I'd stepped off the ride yesterday, but that doesn't appear to be the case.

Last night, when I went to bed I was assaulted by hot flashes; I'm talking waking up drenched in sweat, along with numbness in my right index finger and thumb, numbness in my left foot and the occasional shooting pain down my legs. Let's just say it wasn't my most peaceful slumber to date. Unfortunately, it lasted through today as well.

Because I personified death warmed over, I frantically tried to get my yoga class covered this morning. Literally dialing up at 10:15 with class starting at 10:35. I made it through by sheer stubbornness, although I did have to teach the last 30 minutes just sitting on my mat. Wobbly and weak.

Enough of detailing my litany of physical ailments, as that is very boring. But, if someone else reading this has experienced the same thing, maybe it is helpful to not feel like the only person in the world with a body out of control.

The nature of this disease is simply isolating. The other day, I was talking to my friend who just completed her chemotherapy. We concurred that it is often easier to just stay in the house then make the effort to put on the makeup, wig and/or hat. Easier to shut down.

Today, I finally got to catch up with one of my best friends and hear all the wonderful things that are

162

happening in her life. A nice lengthy phone conversation felt like a luxury. It felt so great to connect. I am looking forward to the time where spending time on the phone and in person is once again the norm. I miss my friends.

Okay, the rollercoaster is cresting. Todd and I just booked our tickets to Australia for September 17th to October 3rd. The light at the end of the tunnel!

Monday, May 24th: Change is the only constant

My primary focus now is to remember to take things day by day. Gratitude. To savor each moment when I feel good, from basking in the San Diego sunshine, enjoying a movie on the couch with Todd, cuddling with Oreo and Jake, to smiling at the commercial for the premiere of *Eclipse* next month. Yes, it makes me smile.

Just as I attempt to enjoy each positive moment, I am trying to remind myself that the hours of feeling fatigued, the numbness in my hands and feet, the new weird red marks on my hands, the waves of depression that inevitably settle in won't last forever. It isn't permanent. Nothing is.

I recall consoling friends who were going through difficult situations to remember that things would get better. I remember others giving me the same advice when I experienced the nadir and felt hopeless. The tide always turns. Really, the only thing we can count on in this lifetime is that nothing is permanent. That you never know what beautiful experience is awaiting you tomorrow. To hold on during the lows in order to ascend to the heights once again.

Today, 10 days out from Round Four, I really still don't feel very well. I'm doing my best to stay optimistic. Yoga, meditation, writing in my journal, staying connected with my friends and family, enjoying nature. Part of me just wants to go to sleep for the next five weeks and wake up and this will all be history.

I do know that this final climb is going to be the most challenging for me. I'm exhausted. I'm extra sensitive and emotional. Prickly. My hearing is more acute. Like a bat. My sense of smell is sharper each day. Like a hound. Call me BatHound.

Tuesday, May 25th: A contest...

For all of you who've told me you weren't comfortable posting comments on the blog: how about voting on the blog? I went out on a limb and opted for a short auburn wig. An alter-ego.

So, let's name her. I'm thinking French and exotic. Brigitte and Chantalle are the front-runners, but I am open to suggestion! Please help me name her! Her maiden voyage on my big bald head is tomorrow morning to teach Pilates.

I am close to 100% today and it feels good. I'm hopeful that the next week continues this trend and I'll be able to take advantage of feeling stronger and be able to do more yoga, do more Pilates, do more walking on the beach. To have the strength to live life on a larger scale and not be held back by these side effects is all I want.

Wednesday, May 26th: Dominique has a fabulous day

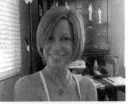

And the winner is...Dominique! Thanks Arch, for your creative vision.

Dominique's inaugural excursion was a smashing success. She taught Pilates, went out to lunch, shopped, and even did some laundry, all in sassy style. Whereas I still feel self-conscious in Sheila or sometimes even in one of the hat-hairs, Dominique is so radically different that I felt liberated.

So, whether it is the fact that I am almost two weeks out from Round Four and physically stronger each day or that life as a redhead is just more exciting, I feel good today. I feel more connected. That vague feeling of isolation is lifting and my mind and heart feel stimulated.

And, I took another step forward in taking my career to the next level. The final piece of the puzzle, you could say. I attended an informational call with Coach U, a life coaching training school. For many years, I've been interested in adding coaching to my arsenal, as a natural extension of teaching yoga and Pilates and seeking to help others. It sounds like an amazing program that won't interrupt my teaching and writing schedule, only complement it.

Why add a coaching credential?

I'd like to help others who have gone through a life-changing crisis, like cancer or AIDS or losing a loved one. I'd like to help pave the way back from darkness to the light. To reconnect with the physical body, the heart and the mind. I'd also like to help motivate those who just feel generally stuck and need encouragement and a plan to implement a professional or personal transformation. Coaching just gives some more structure and tools to the process.

Many people I've encountered have no idea where to start, how to rebuild, how to recreate a life after a crisis. One thing I know is change! If I can share lessons from my experiences, if I can make a difference, if I can heal in some small way, I am fulfilled. Mind, body and spirit.

Now, need to continue working on my own healing.

Thursday, May 27th: Full Moon rising

Based on how I've been feeling the last few days, I can now predict the future. Ha!

Here goes: on the following dates: June 12th through the 24th AND July 3rd to forever...I will be feeling pretty darned good. Please feel free to schedule social visits, attend my yoga classes, and pick up the phone. You may catch glimpses of me around the county, masquerading as Sheila, Dominique, Giselle or Britney, depending upon the day.

The crystal ball says to avoid me June 6th through 12th and June 27th until July 3rd. At all costs. Really, just ask Todd about last week. Visualize a crabby little kid whose summer camp session was canceled and had to stay home and play Monopoly with the parents. Not pretty. Don't be surprised if I don't answer the phone. But do leave me a kind message anyway.

It is so satisfying to have the energy to go meet a friend for lunch, to have the energy to go buy two new tires, to teach yoga, to attend a healing evening filled with several beautiful, strong women. Another good day.

Tonight I attended a very special, energizing event at the home of Victoria Bearden, a talented astrologer in Encinitas. She hosted a Full Moon Manifestation Circle. What is a Full Moon Manifestation Circle you ask?

Essentially, it is an opportunity to write down manifestations you want to create in your life, harness the energy of a group of like-minded positive women, and enjoy a Tibetan bowl meditation culminated by sitting around an outdoor fire pit together and releasing your written card into the fire. Very powerful.

What I found interesting was that I wrote down three manifestations. Nothing on the list had anything to do with breast cancer or health. Nothing. From the beginning of this journey, it never once occurred to me that I was going to die from this disease. Well, okay, maybe once or twice. I'm not afraid of death; I just know it isn't my time yet. Too much to do.

I've got so much that has been incubating as I've been in my I Dream of Jeannie bottle these last months. As I wrote the other day, many of my dreams seem to be crystallizing. I know that my future is incredible and I am on the path to being what I am meant to be, doing what I am meant to do.

Saturday, May 29th: 1st Annual Writer's Block Day

I officially have writer's block today. Check back tomorrow and perhaps my brain will click back to "on."

Sunday, May 30th: Voila!

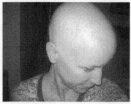

I awoke to discover that I have Monday off! Originally, I was scheduled to teach Pilates at 7:30 a.m. and yoga at noon, but now I've got the entire day free. What a great way to start the day. Not that I don't love teaching, but having two days in a row completely free is a luxury.

Yesterday was rough emotionally. I couldn't shake the dark cloud obscuring all else. My attempts to write both here and on my dusty little novel were fruitless. I ended up putting down quite a bit and then deleting it all. On purpose. The joys of computers. Back in college, I'd have had to tear up the typewritten pages instead of simply hitting one key to obliterate them.

We lounged at the pool this afternoon and soaked up a little sunshine. Slathered with SPF 60 sunscreen of course. Nothing relaxes me more than reading a good book with the sun warming my skin and a cool ocean breeze keeping me from overheating.

I've decided to re-read all of my Hemingway novels. He is my favorite author. I plowed halfway through *The Sun Also Rises* at the pool. Hemingway captures Paris perfectly and makes me so nostalgic for the time when I was lucky enough to live there. Nobody can capture the romanticism of writing, drinking and eating in Paris, of living in the moment. Nobody can elicit the same emotions.

A Moveable Feast is next. Actually, it is my favorite, so I should save it for last after I revisit *For Whom the Bell Tolls*. Not my favorite. Importantly, I can totally escape into Hemingway's world, leaving my issues behind. And, he motivates me to write. The more I read his work, the more I am able to flow within mine. I'll finish that novel yet.

In terms of milestones for today, 25 days remain until my last day of chemotherapy. Three and one-half weeks. When I glance in the rearview mirror, I am amazed that it is almost the five-month mark from the fateful date I found the lump. Is fateful a word?

After the last chemo, I've got a break for two or three weeks, then seven weeks of daily radiation, so August appears to be the true end to this ordeal. I actually still don't understand the radiation. If the chemotherapy is assassinating all the cells in my body, wouldn't it kill the ones surrounding the lump removal site? Isn't radiation a little bit redundant? Does my body really need any more collateral damage than it has already received?

I've been very anxious that I am developing lymphedema in my right arm. I may have overdone my Pilates on Friday and my right chest, back, deltoid and arm feel heavy and swollen. My underarm is still totally numb and the inside of my upper arm is numb too, so it is hard to ascertain what is happening.

The road to recovery is rough. I'm trying to maintain some daily activity, but when my legs refuse to budge, walking is a challenge. I was planning on practicing flow yoga, but I cannot put any weight on my right arm until it feels normal again. I'll do my range of motion and flexibility exercises, but it is so frustrating to be unable to really move and get the endorphins flowing.

So much restriction. So many rules. I can't wait until my body can do what my mind desires it to do. Patience has always been a major issue for me. I attribute that primarily to my French heritage. French- Corsican heritage. It is in my blood to be impatient, impetuous and passionate.

Cancer requires the complete opposite set of emotional skills and although I began practicing yoga in 1999, I am not equipped to calmly proceed through the maze that is cancer treatment. Too bad this cancer didn't wait about 20 more years to hit me.

Chapter 6: June

Tuesday, June 1st: 23 days to go

I will laze around like a lump all weekend. Todd and I are going to Napa on Thursday and I need to feel fabulous! A romantic few days, staying at a winery in a beautiful loft converted from a barn, surrounded by vines. Motivation to rest now.

Yesterday was a great Memorial Day holiday. My newly engaged friend Angie and her fiancé Darin surprised us with an impromptu visit. The last few times Angie visited were dominated by the head-shaving party, the liver biopsy and bringing snacks to me as I was housebound with the evil drain. It was wonderful to actually have a social rendezvous instead! We hit the beach, enjoyed a delicious dinner at Via Italia and relaxed and caught up. Fabulous.

On Thursday I have Chemo Round Five, which signals that it is officially THREE WEEKS until the last round of chemotherapy. Pretty amazing that there really is an end to this portion of the journey. In sight.

I've been practicing more yoga at home, specifically targeted to Yoga for Cancer Recovery. I've been utilizing the training I completed back in April. Although I miss attending class, at this point I have to accept that my energy is low and adjust my practice accordingly.

On the physical side, I feel weaker since the last round of chemotherapy. My legs are consistently fatigued, sore and generally not my own. I guess the cumulative effect is weighing me down. My right arm and shoulder still feel swollen and tight and I am praying that it isn't lymphedema. Please, please, please no!

Emotionally, I can envision the light at the end of the tunnel and am excited for a true countdown. Radiation just feels like it will be an afterthought after chemo. I hope I'm not being naive! My patience is at an end. Did I really just say that? What patience? Ha. Dare I dream of a day when I return to a regular schedule? The "hold" that has been in effect will be lifted and I can start sowing some of the seeds planted during these last months.

Twenty-three days to go...

Wednesday, June 2nd: Chemo-Eve Number Five

The Tang-orange bag is packed. Again. Ready to head to Scripps.

Gossip magazines: Check.
Ipod: Check.
$400 anti-nausea medication: Check.
Incredible soft blanket from Dreamy: Check.
Crunchy cinnamon sugar pita chips from Trader Joe's: Check.

Today turned out to be a good day. I continued to feel off-kilter this morning, but the lovely Christy treated me to an hour-long reflexology session at De la Sole Reflexology Spa in Del Mar. Delicious! The studio is completely Zen, with big overstuffed chairs, soft lighting and peaceful music. Sixty minutes of a head massage, arm and hand massage and a fabulous foot reflexology massage. I accessed that blessed space between sleep and consciousness and left feeling relaxed and refreshed. I highly recommend it!

I'm flying on my mandatory steroids. My 6 p.m. Pilates Reformer class benefitted from the energy this evening! Even though I resemble GI Jane, I'm looking forward to teaching yoga in the morning before chemo. Can't wait for the hair to return...

The day was capped off by a fantastic dinner delivery from the sweet, generous Lori. Yum. It has been such a gift to have dinner delivered over these last few months. It simplifies the day and alleviates the burden on Todd. Thank you. Thank you. Thank you.

No big lessons today, but I'm sure epiphanies are percolating. Day by day.

Friday, June 4th: Five down, One to go!

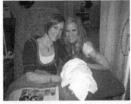

I cannot believe that I've completed five rounds of chemotherapy. Fifteen weeks! One more to go. Ever. It hasn't quite sunk in yet. Bring on June 24th!

Dominique graced my big bald head on yesterday's round, which took place in the fancy new Chemo Lounge with a bird's-eye view of the Torrey Pines Golf Course. Nikke was wonderful company and I appreciated her being there with me for acupuncture and chemo. Todd arrived for the final hour and ride home.

Interestingly, a woman named Sheila who was there for her first treatment came by my chair to compliment me on Dominique. I informed her that I had another wig named Sheila! She is going to meet with Patti the amazing wig lady on Tuesday. Sheila is going to name one of her wig's Claire. Ahhh, the tangled webs we weave.

Last night, I lay down at 6 p.m. and didn't wake until 8:30 the next morning! Wow. No nausea again, thanks to Lois, the magical acupuncturist. I am convinced that I haven't had any major issues with nausea because of her skill with the needles.

Frogs Yoga this morning. Today's feedback was that I was feisty, which means that the steroids were in full effect. I love the Frogs Yoga Friday crew. Such beautiful energy. Après-class I enjoyed the requisite lululemon visit. And purchases. Who can resist? Fabulous people, fabulous clothes! Didn't I learn that steroid induced shopping is dangerous when Kim was visiting?

I'm thrilled to announce that I will be teaching a weekly Yoga for Cancer Therapy class at the lululemon store during August. This class will be specifically tailored for all types of cancer patients and those recovering from cancer treatment. Thereafter, I plan on starting an ongoing weekly class in North County. I cannot wait to commence down this path.

Treatment-wise: I've got my CT scan scheduled for July 15th. We'll see if that pesky spot continues to lurk on my liver, whether it has shrunk or if it is gone. My vote is disappearance. Follow up with the oncologist on July 23rd. Seven weeks of radiation treatment starts around that time and I'm also supposed to start on the five-year Tamoxifin drugs. Not sure if the Tamoxifin and I will work out.

Silver lining: the chemotherapy portion of this ride is almost over.

174

Sunday, June 6th: Napping with Oreo

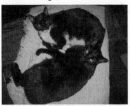

Round Five Thursday. Check.

Oreo's Round Three Steroid shot yesterday. Check.
Mama Cat and Oreo nap together. Check.

Monday, June 7th: Round Five better than Four

Thus far, Round Five greatly exceeds Round Four. No huge bloated Uncle Fester head. No extreme muscle pain. No useless, exhausted limbs.

Actually, today was quite productive. I'm in my element when I check items off of my to-do list. Confirmed that my accountant filed my taxes, yes, they were late but hey, I figured I had a good excuse for an extension. Good news is that I actually got a refund. Direct to the Great Barrier Reef fund.

The highlight of my day was a complimentary facial. Free facial. No charge for cancer patients. How wonderful is that? Facelogic Spa in Encinitas offers free facials for cancer patients every other month. They donate their time and talent to give others going through challenging times some much-needed pampering. From the moment I walked into the soothing environment, I felt special. After my appointment with Mareli, my skin felt like buttah!

Upon arriving home, the lovely Bonnie dropped off a tasty dinner of sweet potatoes and salmon. The sweet potatoes were so yummy that I stuffed myself beyond the brim. Will I ever learn to stop gorging? Too good to resist!

I plan on taking it easy this week in order to fully recuperate so that I go into Round Six as strong as possible. We are looking at days people, days. Seventeen days. Then, no more chemo ever. No. More. Chemo. Ever. Again.

I wish I were feeling more articulate so I could express what's brewing inside. I'm afraid that my brain is rather floaty and loose right now. Perhaps later this week, some of these realizations and lessons will solidify enough to be documented.

Wednesday, June 9th: Meditation, Music and Ben & Jerry

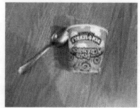

Diverse experiences can alter one's mood, don't you think? All in unique ways. I am a different person tonight from this morning thanks to meditation, music and B&J's.

This morning, I awoke with my customary Day-Six-Post-Chemo-Irritable-Witch-From-Hell hat securely in place. Just like a newborn comes screaming out into the world, I awoke howling and red-faced. Well, maybe not red-faced, but you get the picture.

Claire's Issue du Jour: Cooped up for too long. Unable to exercise in any way that really felt like working out. Unable to prevent my muscles' gradual atrophy from head to toe. Unable to focus my brain in a satisfying manner for more than 10 minutes.

Recognizing my condition, I chose to correct it. Much to Jake and Oreo's horror, I screeched a few times. They prefer me quiet and cuddly. I then spouted off in my Twilight journal. It is almost full and then I can start on the New Moon journal. Working through the tin journal collection that I received for Christmas from Todd's mom who is acquainted with my obsession.

I gathered my dignity and taught Pilates, which always cheers me up. I love my 8:30 a.m. crew: such positive energy and simply fun. Afterwards, I did a mild reformer workout for myself to get the blood flowing.

Prior to class, I'd sent out an S.O.S. to my friend Stephanie's husband, Mike, who is a healer and teacher of meditation. Meditation Emergency! I needed a house call, pronto.

I may have mentioned a few hundred times that I have trouble meditating unless I physically exhaust myself first. Vinyasa yoga is meditation for me. Without the asana practice, however, I cannot calm the overactive brain. Since my practice is virtually non-existent due to the chemo and my right arm not being quite right yet, I haven't meditated. I desperately need it. My goal is to meditate daily, without any need for yoga or any other physical exertion. A lofty aim. Enter Mike!

Mike, like all gifted teachers, reminded me that I already know how to meditate. I don't have to practice yoga first. I just had to sit down, close my eyes and DO IT. Random thoughts popped up, anything from not having time to see the Great Barrier Reef to a craving for mashed potatoes to wondering if I should move my foot because it had fallen dead asleep. He guided me through what I assumed was about 15 minutes and it was actually 35 minutes! Calmed, centered and ready for a nap. I have a plan for tomorrow morning's solo meditation. Thank you Mike!

Later the same day, on my way to teach my lovely 6 p.m. Pilates crew, I hit the radio bonanza. I actually sang to Incubus and Rage Against the Machine all the way to Frogs and had to sit in my car to listen to Chris Cornell's "Like a Stone." A little Pearl Jam "Black" and Stone Temple Pilots completed my fabulous set. Thank you 91X. I've got the musical taste of a teenage boy (teenage boy in the 90s) and hearing some of my favorites, all in a row, just lifted me up. Music is such a transporter and healer for me. Different than the meditation, but just as effective to shift my mood.

And, finally, the pint of Ben & Jerry's Cinnamon Buns ice cream sent me over the edge. Can you say sugar high? One side-effect from the chemotherapy is that often nothing tastes cold enough. Even putting ice in water fails to cool it beyond lukewarm for me.

Thus, I've been craving ice cream and I'm not an ice cream person. I like my sweets to be baked. Cookies, cake, cupcakes, brownies: that's my MO. Cancer Claire prefers ice cream and frozen yogurt. The ice cream feels just chilly enough. So refreshing in fact that I looked down and I'd polished off the pint. I guess all that singing rendered my throat extra dry.

Tonight, I feel great. Choosing to take action and ask for help with the meditation was all I needed to start me in the right direction. Tomorrow, I will wake up with a smile.

Thursday, June 10th: Ambassador challenge

Rollercoaster...whoo hoo hoo hoo. Rode the Cinnamon Bun ice cream high until 1 p.m. today.

I woke up and meditated, with the assistance of Jake and Oreo. It wasn't pretty. My mind was flying all over the place, but I persevered, observed the million thoughts per minute, and when I opened my eyes, 20 minutes had elapsed. Success. Practice and persistence. First thing in the morning may not be the best time for me because I wake up raring to get started and that makes clearing the mind a little tough. I'll experiment tomorrow.

Drum roll...big news: I am officially registered with CoachU, the leading global provider of coach training programs! I'm enrolled and ready to start in July. I love school. I am so excited!

The program is provided via teleclasses and one of my initial classes is at 6 a.m. on Thursday mornings. For some reason, Todd finds this amusing. I taught a 5:30 a.m. yoga class for three years. 5:30 AM! I used to do Outside Sales for an "East Coast" company that didn't care about people on the "West Coast" and routinely scheduled mind-numbing conference calls at 5 and 6 a.m. So, there is no reason why I cannot roll from bed to desk, armed with major caffeine and sit on the phone and computer at 6 a.m. As long as Skype isn't involved, I'm safe in my Hello Kitty pajamas.

My energy dipped dramatically this afternoon. The cats are so happy that I've seen the light about numerous daily naps. It is so weird how I can feel fine one moment and the next I absolutely must lay down. Boom, no warning. It is part of what makes me nervous about going to yoga or other classes: the fear of collapsing in the middle of the class. Like the Energizer Bunny. Only two weeks until my final chemo so, I expect my energy to return in July.

Just in time for lululemon ambassador month! We had our first official ambassador meeting this evening and I was thrilled to meet some of the other ambassadors for the first time. What a line-up! From Tim Miller of the Ashtanga Yoga Center, to Shannon of Pure Barre La Costa, to Gina the Soccer Coach/Runner/PhD candidate, to Robert "Mr. Kettlebell", to Dejinira the amazing Personal Trainer and Zumba Master, it is quite a group. Add Dre, Natalie and Laura from lulu and it was an inspiring evening. I am honored to be part of this group.

Lots of brainstorming occurred and we agreed that it was a fabulous idea for the ambassadors and the lululemon Carlsbad community to have a July challenge where we all get out of our comfort zones and run around taking everybody else's classes. It will be exhilarating to join this challenge and highly entertaining to watch yogis swing kettlebells and runners get on a little zumba and...the possibilities are endless. I can't wait.
But, for tonight, my energy has once again elapsed.

Night night.

Saturday, June 12th: Rollercoaster hitting the valley

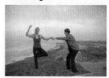

Feeling wobbly, just like I did in this photo balancing on one foot in the freezing iceplant. Thank goodness for Laura saving me from a tumble off the cliff.

Sadly, my rollercoaster seems to be hovering in the bottom of the dip. Head on up, up, up! My energy levels are so low that I felt totally woozy and almost fell over at the cat house at Petco this morning. This nosedive began yesterday afternoon and won't abate. Is that the same timeframe when the white and red blood cell counts hit their lowest?

How does this make me feel? Two options for you: mild flu when you ache all over, your stomach is jumpy and you just want grilled cheese and tomato soup. Or, you went dancing last night and it seemed like a good idea to have that third apple martini, or margarita or whatever potent concoction that would have seduced you. Either option yields the same result: must stay horizontal. Very disappointing! This unpredictability really bothers me.

Okay, the bright side: this will be the last dip I'll have knowing that I'll get knocked down again after my final chemo on June 24th. Thereafter, only ascension. Never again. If by some terrible chance I have a recurrence, I refuse to do chemo again. This I know for sure.

Sunday, June 13th: And up we go!

What a difference a day makes. I awoke feeling much better than I have since before the last round. How refreshing! I must confess that I slept until 10 a.m. Perhaps sleeping for almost 12 hours healed me.

San Diego has been dominated by June Gloom for the last few weeks so, I was overjoyed that the sun decided to shine today. Sunshine and legs that didn't feel like cement blocks! To celebrate, we went for a walk at the lagoon. Such a beautiful, tranquil environment, graced with sun-dappled trees, graceful egrets and other birds. It felt great to be outside, to be active and to be off the couch.

181

Gratitude has played a huge part in this journey. Gratitude for the love and support that I have received. Gratitude that I've tolerated the treatment well, for the most part. I've saved every single card, email and note that I've received since this all began in January. Today, I spent some time re-reading some of them.

I feel so blessed for the kind words, the well-wishes, the prayers, and the sentiment. It is so uplifting to revisit all of them. It gives me renewed energy and faith to make it through the next weeks of chemo and the seven weeks of radiation.

My plans for providing Yoga for Cancer Recovery are falling into place. This week I should have a schedule for the month-long free series of classes that I will offer at lululemon for patients and survivors of all types of cancer. We plan to create all kinds of resources. Exciting!

Three days until Napa!

Tuesday, June 15th: Getting emotional

This week is progressing well thus far. I'm very excited to escape to Napa Valley on Thursday! Nothing like getting out of town for a few days, especially somewhere as beautiful as Napa. We get to stay in the middle of a vineyard! Talk about heaven.

So, for some reason I am crying often these days.

This morning, I cried when I made my appointment with the Radiation Oncologist. Mid-July is full of doctor's appointments again. It may sound strange, but having chemo every three weeks was kind of a nice hiatus compared to the testing phase prior to it. At that point, Todd wanted to buy a frequent flier parking pass because we were at Scripps so often. As did all my friends who accompanied me to various probings.

I go in for a CT-Scan of my abdomen on July 15th to see if the liver spot has changed. All this chemo poison should've knocked it out if it were anything other than a cyst or birthmark. I am staying positive on the liver spot! If it is bad news, Todd and I are hitting France and Italy before Australia! Travel time...

The following day, I see my Radiation Oncologist for a tattooing of my right boob where they will direct the radiation beam. Every single day, five days a week for seven weeks. Yes, my poor right boob. Darn! I've never wanted a tattoo, never wanted a permanent mark on my body and now I've got no choice. Scars and tattoos are unwelcome, uninvited reminders of the big C.

And, more daily crying for Oreo and his cancer. I can really see him slowing down. The vet told me that with his type of cancer, it is usually a matter of months. I hope he holds on! His last steroid shot didn't seem to be as effective as the first two. At night, he has developed an unfortunate pattern of howling at the top of his lungs while jumping up onto the bed. He purrs for five minutes, settles in just long enough for me to return to sleep, and then hops off. Repeat. Several times. Not good for Todd and my REM sleep let me tell you.

For some reason, Oreo can sleep uninterrupted for several hours during the day. He snoozed right through the earthquake last night. Hmmmm...funny how that works. Maybe I should wake him up repeatedly all day? That would show him! Seriously though, he resembles a little old man these days. I've had him for nine years, so it is a challenging process to begin letting him go. Hopefully not anytime soon.

Time to go teach yoga. That blessed relief from thinking about me, me, me and giving to others. Without the gift of teaching, I may have given up hope.

Wednesday, June 16th: Napa-Eve

Here I am, eve-ing it up again. I am excited to leave for Napa first thing in the morning! I'm packed and ready to go. Todd is already up in San Francisco so it feels like I'm flying off to meet my lover in an exotic locale. Sunshine, a room amongst the vines, wine, delicious food and Todd: I cannot wait! Will it be Dominique or Sheila stepping off that plane?

Today was fantastic. One of the best days I've had in a while. I taught two Pilates classes and the new Yoga for Healthy Backs class at Bindu Yoga. I enjoyed a leisurely lunch with my dear friend Zoe at one of my favorite restaurants, St. Tropez. We've both been so busy that actually having the time to just eat lunch and catch up seemed decadent. She's one of those people that you simply feel good being around.

On days like today, I don't feel like I have cancer at all. Well, except for a few choice moments wrestling with the wigs, but that is another story. I taught, I went to meetings, I got in a workout on the Reformer, I went to lunch, I packed for a really romantic trip: in other words I was fully engaged in my life and my day. Sometimes, throughout this whole ride, I've felt half-alive and numb. It was a gift to feel like Full-blown CLAIRE today.

Friday, June 18th: Napa!

Reynolds Winery, the home of Burt Reynolds the charming orange cat who loved me. Fantastic! Lucky cat!

Glorious weather, unbelievable scenery, perfect company.

184

Next stop, a winding drive up Spring Mountain to Pride Winery. We didn't have an appointment, but I guess we looked trustworthy so they granted us entrance! We didn't just taste, our guide Russ took us through the caves and gave us a barrel tasting. He allowed me to hold the "thief" that removes the 2008 Cabernet straight out of the barrel. It was delicious. Russ also gave us a glass of Chardonnay to take up to the picnic tables that came complete with a panoramic view off of Spring Mountain. We devoured four different types of cheeses from the Cheese Board in Berkeley and fresh baguettes. Who needs anything else?

Two more wineries. Feeling warm and happy.

Lymphedema and a swollen right arm, but I'm praying that goes away. It is a little better today, but I'm very distressed.

We encountered another kitty on the street last night who wasn't as fortunate as the winery cat and got her a can of food. Someone had shaved half her body, she was painfully thin and beaten up. But she was a sweetheart, purred when I petted her and was grateful for an easy dinner. If we were in San Diego, I'd have brought her home. I'm praying someone else will.

Okay, time to transform into a glamorous blonde wine taster!! Darioush, here we come

Sunday, June 20th: Lymphedema ruins everything

I am attempting to recuperate from a scary incident that marred our magical Napa trip. My arm continued to balloon in Napa, to the point that by Saturday morning, my right wrist bone had disappeared and my forearm rivaled Popeye's. Only a small percentage of those who have breast cancer surgeries will develop lymphedema. It looks like I qualify for this group.

What is it? Well, the surgeon removes several lymph nodes to see if the cancer has spread, thus compromising your lymphatic system. Forever. For some, there are no long-term repercussions. For others, fluid pools in places such as your breast, arm, hand and fingers. It is "incurable, painful and sometimes leads to complications." Flying can trigger it.

Yesterday morning, I was freaking out and called the doctor to see if there were any preventative measures prior to boarding the plane to return home. The on-call oncologist told me not to get on the plane and to go to a local emergency room for an ultrasound, as there was danger I could have a blood clot. Huh? Not exactly news I wanted to hear. I wanted to come home. He emphatically stated that he did not recommend that I do that, but if I did to go straight to Urgent Care from the airport. Do not pass go. Do not collect $100. It was not the most comforting of phone calls.

The entire flight home was dominated by thoughts of having an aneurysm on the plane. Comas, brain damage, heart damage, death: you name it. Nobody mentioned the threat of blood clots from lymphedema.

The Lymphedema Association says you can NEVER do a lot of things like: get blood pressure taken on that arm, have blood drawn, get cut or scratched, **get a bug bite**: love this one, what do I do here? "Excuse me Mr. Bee, can you please sting my left arm instead?" NEVER lift more than 15 pounds, avoid alcohol, don't go in a sauna or hot tub, etc.

The most troubling aspect is the potential of having to wear an extremely uncomfortable sleeve each and every time I exercise and fly or if it worsens, all the time. And, the lymphedema specialist I met back in March told me that wearing the sleeve during flying may or may not help. Nobody seems to have any true statistics. Well, I wore the custom-fitted sleeve for most of the flight to Utah in May. It was painfully uncomfortable, not to mention hideously ugly. Imagine orthopedic hose from knuckle to shoulder. Not exactly what I'd like to wear as I teach yoga or workout myself. It would be one thing if I lived in Alaska and was always in long sleeves!

How is that going to work for me as a yoga teacher in sunny San Diego? The doctor yesterday also told me that until the swelling is completely gone that I couldn't teach, much less practice, in the heat where I teach about half of my classes. So, there is a real impact on my career.

I was really feeling optimistic and positive. My last chemo is this week. There is a light at the end of the tunnel. Many of the side effects I've endured would disappear by next month. Imagine: hair! Energy! Regular workouts! Fiber! Now, I feel angry, upset, devastated at how this could impact me. I'm sure I'll reach a place where I'm able to feel positive and overcome it. But, I'm not there yet.

Tuesday, June 22nd: Pumps suck

Today I was treated with a lymphedema pump that crushed my arm for about 30 to 40 minutes to try to drain the lymphatic fluid out of the areas where it is pooling. When this sleeve was removed, it looked like a chef had been pumping my arm with 20 little waffle irons. I'm now trussed up with three ace bandages, reminiscent of the Michelin Man. I must keep the bandages on overnight and pray, pray, pray that the swelling subsides.

After spending three, yes three, hours with the Lymphedema Specialist, I have "mild" lymphedema. It is a permanent, chronic condition that if left untreated, can result in a big, fat, hard sausage-arm. Think the Elephant Man. And, not Ganesha. Now, the goal is to reduce the swelling over the next few weeks with three times per week sessions of lymphatic massage and the giant waffle iron sleeve. If it fails to shrink in the next few weeks, it will permanently be bigger than the other arm.

What does this mean? The good news is I don't have to wear a compression sleeve daily. Huge relief. I'll have to monitor every single workout, what weight I pick up: from a grocery bag to my cat, as well as "vigorous activity"...whatever the hell that means.

If I start to see swelling, I can wrap my arm overnight with the ace bandages. This, by the way, is incredibly uncomfortable. I will have to wrap the arm every time I fly. Forever. That doesn't seem like such a huge deal compared to the day-to-day vigilance. Pilot lessons may be out, however.

Time will tell what will affect this. I'm convinced that the swelling must come down because I refuse to have a fat elbow and forearm forever. Time will tell what will exacerbate this. I'm going to do my stretches and slowly build the strength up in this arm and just pray that the wrapping will be on rare occasions. I WILL get my pre-cancer arm and body back.

On that note, I also had my recommended consultation with the head of plastic surgery at Scripps to discuss options if I want corrective breast surgery after radiation. There are some options, but the best news all day (sadly) is that although fat transfer is very popular these days, I'm too lean to harvest any fat from. After all the bread, cheese and pain au chocolat from Napa, that is indeed my silver lining.

Wednesday, June 23rd: As the arm shrinks...

Chemo Eve. I'm shifting my focus to celebratory: chemotherapy is almost over forever! This time, I know I'll have my downtime, but it is finite. Thereafter, I will continue to get strong, rebuild my muscles and bones and develop some hair on this egg-like head.

Thank you everyone for the offers of fat harvesting: at this rate I could build boobs the size of Dolly Parton. I only need about a golf-ball amount so; perhaps everyone could write an essay on why they have the richest, plumpest fat and why their fat would make the best boob filler. Apparently, belly fat works very well. I don't know how I'd feel about having someone's butt fat on my chest. Keep that in mind. Thank you for making me laugh.

After sleeping, or shall I say attempting to sleep, with the Michelin Man arm, I gingerly unwrapped all of the bandages. Nervous, eager and hesitant to look at my arm, I nonetheless glanced down. Was this how Michael Jackson felt each and every time he got a new nose job?

I'm happy to report that the swelling has definitely subsided a lot. I can see my wrist again and the wrinkles on the inside of my elbows. The upper arm surrounding my elbow is still puffy, but not quite as puffy. You can see some bone at the tip. Hurray!! I will continue with the exercises and wrapping my arm before bed and pray that the remaining bloat will disappear. The therapist said we'll continue therapy for a few weeks and by then it should reach optimal size so, fingers crossed. I'm now feeling optimistic that I won't have an elephant arm.

I have an awesome "Chemo Graduation Day" T-shirt to wear tomorrow, courtesy of Anaise--thank you very much! It is perfect. Depending upon how I feel after chemo, I'm craving Wine Steals pizza. Celebration!!

Thursday, June 24th: Chemo Graduation Day

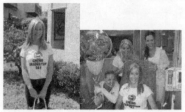

Everyone at Scripps loved my Chemo Graduation T-shirt! It was absolutely perfect, thank you again Anaise! Thanks to Meredith, Anne and Rachel for sharing some of the afternoon with me. The last afternoon ever in the Chemo Lounge for me.

It hasn't really hit me yet that I am done with the worst part of treatment. It is finished. Behind me. Never have to go again. Now my hair can start growing back. As I lost five more eyebrow hairs yesterday, that is a good thing. I'm starting to look like the lady who worked at Fairfax Hospital cafeteria with fully drawn-on brows!

Now, it is time to move forward!! To focus on building new strength, stamina, and getting my arm under control. Coach U starts next week so I can begin the journey of rounding out my career and add Life Coach to my resume. Officially, that is! I'm looking forward to getting back to a regular teaching schedule, to planning the lululemon Yoga for Cancer Recovery collaboration we've set up for August.

And, most importantly, to have this cancer fade into the background. Never forgotten, but no longer the star of the show. I've got too much to live for, too much to do, too many people to love. And, for now, the Sandman is beckoning.

Monday, June 28th: Rough skies

Not up for writing, but...

Let's just say that while I am happy that the chemo phase is over, this is the darkest and most challenging recuperation phase thus far. Right now, I cannot visualize the light at the end of the tunnel. I know it is there, but just out of reach. Maybe when I wake up tomorrow...

Tuesday, June 29th: Nemesis

Well, this final recovery from chemotherapy isn't quite what I had envisioned. I was fully prepared to have wobbly legs like a colt, to need lots of rest, to take all my meds and herbs, to rinse my mouth out with warm salt water, and all the other tricks I've acquired along the way. Little did I know that I'd be trapped in the house like I was with the godforsaken surgery drain. This time, however, I am bandaged up like a mummy, knowing that the bandages will play an as yet undetermined role in my future.

Part of the nightmare of this last week is embodied in the lymphedema specialist. You know when you meet someone for the first time and yet you recognize them? You click? As if you've known each other before? Well, with M, it was the opposite. Her gaze sent a chill down my spine. She is not here to help or heal; in fact, her words and actions have had the opposite effect.

Today was the last day of her negative influence. I know this may be surprising, but I am a wimp with personal confrontation. Nonetheless, I put on my big girl panties this afternoon and called to tell the office that I wasn't comfortable working with her and wanted another therapist. They instantly obliged me, no questions asked.

So, what was the problem with this person who made me cry in the office not once, but twice?

Here are some of her words, delivered impatiently to me over the last week:

"You have a lot of anger issues over your breast cancer and you just need to get over it,"

"Stop being so dramatic," (when I saw my arm after the pump was removed)

"This is a permanent condition and you just need to deal with it,"

"Just get used to wrapping yourself in bandages, maybe daily for the rest of your life."

Mind you, this woman doesn't know me. At all. Knows nothing about me, my attitudes, my strengths, my weaknesses. Except that I just finished Round Six of chemo and have developed lymphedema. Perhaps a bit of compassion?

Besides her remarks, her other behavior has been inappropriate and wrong. Last week, she showed me how to do lymphatic self-massage. This is when it got weird: we are in a small room, with the curtain drawn. First, she pulls her sleeve down to rub her collarbone and shoulder. Okay. The next thing you know, she whips off her shirt and is standing there in her bra and pants, massaging her chest and arm. I was extremely uncomfortable. Why did she feel the need to doff her shirt? Then, she grabs a roll around her waist and says how now that she is 58 she has love handles. WHAT???

So, why was I afraid to call the physical therapy department and request a different therapist? Isn't that interesting? Do I care if I hurt this woman's feelings? No, not at all. Is it more about being uncomfortable if I see her in the department and she knows I requested not to work with her anymore? Maybe. I find it interesting that they made the switch with No Questions Asked. I am excited to have a new therapist.

So, my world has been small and unpleasant this week. I am processing, going through it and am hoping this will be just another speed bump in my rearview mirror. That the pump/bandage 24/7 therapy will be over soon. That I can focus on healing my whole body, heart and mind. That next week is new, fresh and I feel strong again.

Wednesday, June 30th: Cat naps

Quiet times. Me and the kitties. Sleeping, napping, lying about or eating. Oreo and Jake are quite pleased that I've seen the light and am sharing their usual schedule, without pesky interruptions like leaving the house or interacting with other humans. Oreo seems to be slowing down and just wants to be curled up close to me. So, I guess there is a silver lining in being housebound.

I'm shocked at how exhausted I am. I've been drinking my fresh vegetable juice and popping all types of antioxidants and herbs in the desperate hope that they'll infuse my limbs with some vitality. Or, at least I won't get winded dragging myself from the couch to the bed! Give me my legs back!

Tomorrow. Tomorrow is a big day! I have two major appointments.

At 8:30 a.m., I meet a new lymphedema specialist. Knowing that I have a new therapist, who will hopefully be nice to me, despite ironing my arm in the compression machine and wrapping me up like a mummy, is encouraging. I hope to get some answers: such as when my arm will be back to normal, when I can do Down Dog and whether I'll have to wear a sleeve when I do it, how to prevent another flare-up and all that good stuff.

The big event, and trust me, as only someone who has been cooped up in the house for seven nights can say, this is epic: I have an 11 a.m. date to see *Eclipse* with Kirsten. Go Team Edward. *Eclipse* was my favorite book and I can't wait to see it play out on the big screen.

Anticipation…I wonder if I'll be able to sleep tonight? Not kidding.

Chapter 7: July

Friday, July 2nd: Adventures in mail-order

San Diegans are outraged at the extreme gray weather blanketing our fine city. June Gloom is over and it should be sunny beach weather. Although I would usually be marching at the head of the Sunshine Parade, the gloom has been the perfect setting for me. I've been a diluted version of myself: Shadow of Claire. I'm ready to remove the dimmer switch and shine very soon.

I'll share the most amusing moment of the entire week, thus lending you some insight into my week: the delivery of my Ovation Cell Therapy treatment. According to the radio and a few other personal testimonials, this concoction will grow my hair back thicker and fuller than ever before. If you remember my hair, not a big challenge.

When the doorbell rang, I was inside on the couch or bed, take your pick. Since I was in my full bald splendor complete with Michelin Man Mummy Arm, I chose not to answer the door. Call me vain. As soon as I was certain the FedEx man had departed, I yanked the door open, snatched the package with my mummy arm and scuttled back into the cave with my prize.

I've been carefully washing my bald head with the shampoo and then massaging the Cell Therapy Treatment in the shower. I'm saving the conditioner portion of the ritual for when I actually have some hairs to put it on. I'm sure those follicles are getting fired up and ready to sprout out long, curly golden locks. Ha. I can dream right? Hell, they can come in silver and curly as long as they come in fast and will respond to Blonde Dye!

I've had the attention span of a grasshopper this week. Hopefully, this isn't a side effect of slathering my scalp with the Ovation gunk. No ability to focus on completing anything that I need to complete, no sustained effort or if I am honest, no sustained interest in anything. I've just not had the energy to do anything. Physically or mentally. Perhaps it isn't just lymphatic fluid in my arm, but brain fluid has drained down to give me a fat elbow?

I did read some of my early blog entries from January and February. Wow, a lifetime ago. Tests, diagnoses, surgery, the drain, and so on. One thing that shines through is the amazing love and support that I've received from friends, family, students and even those that I didn't know.

Once treatment is finished and I feel officially "healed", it will be interesting to sit down and actually read the entire journey: I need a title: **Bridget Jones Diary Meets Claire's Right Boob?**

Sunday, July 4th: Little hairs...

Okay, this is getting ridiculous. Where is the sun? My toes are painted patriotic blue, my bikini is orange, and my giant pink hat that adequately hides my big bald head was securely in place. Slathered on sunscreen. New *InStyle* magazine. Lovely sarong, that I forgot how to tie...I need another lesson.

No sun. And, not only is there no sun, it is cold and breezy! Absolutely unacceptable.

So here I sit, hunched over the computer at the peak of what should be a sunny 4th of July. Harrumph. We're going to take out the beach cruisers later, but I'm not sure how wise that is as my hat and hat-hair might blow off in the bitter, cold wind. The last time my hat was pulled off wasn't pretty and I'd prefer to avoid that trauma. Maybe I can tie it on with something?

I am feeling better! Thank goodness! Day 10 after the final chemotherapy treatment and I'm excited to usher in a new era. All of the yucky side effects are starting to fade, one by one.

Emotionally, I feel rather disconnected from most of my friends and the studios where I teach. I just haven't been there fully for so long. I am eager to rebuild a sense of regularity where I teach when I'm scheduled, when I can talk to my friends and make plans that aren't centered around treatment, where things feel more reciprocal. There is a melancholy sense that I've been on ice for six months as everyone else has moved forward. I hope to find synchronicity soon.

On a positive note, some new hairs are sprouting on my head. Not the little half-inch stubble, but actual hairs! There are three in particular that have caught Todd's and my attention. These three, count them, three hairs are about two inches long and appear to have just sprung up. So, if all of them start budding at two inches, I'll be sporting a pixie in no time.

I swore I'd never have a pixie again, but I guess the lesson here is that there is no never or always. The term "pixie haircut" brings up a deep wound between my mother and me. I don't think I've ever forgiven her for it. When I was eight years old, she lured me to the hairdresser for a "trim" and I exited that salon with a pixie. Mind you, I was a gangly little kid and the only feminine feature was my hair. Shorn, I looked like a little boy. Much to my chagrin

197

To be fair, my Mom was probably sick and tired of attempting to brush through the rat's nest that was my long, waist-length hair. We were living in Nairobi at the time and I must admit that I was quite a tomboy. I was always playing outside and if I recall correctly, I wasn't a huge fan of the bathtub or taking my hair out of pigtails. No pink ribbons for me. Traumatized, I vowed never to have short hair again. I succeeded except for an unfortunate haircut and perm combo in high school, but that is another story.

So come on, *grow* little hairs! Grow, multiply, becoming abundant! I'm letting go of absolutes like *never* and *always*…and not just with the hair. I'm ready to reclaim my life, starting with the pixie renaissance.

Monday, July 5th: Back to school!

Back to reality! I feel like a little kid who just returned to school after a long summer away from all her favorite people. What an awesome day! I am pooped.

The morning began at Bindu Yoga in Del Mar, where some of my students from other studios came in and tried the studio for the first time. Lovely energy, lovely class! Then, I headed over to Sculpt Fusion Yoga and was thrilled to see several of my regular students again. It was a familiar homecoming and I couldn't be happier. The workday ended at Pilates with my strong, lovely regulars Leslie and Katharine. How can teaching be so much fun?

Unfortunately, my hand swelled up yesterday and again today. I've been bandaging nightly, but I cannot sleep. Last night, tormented by the bondage, I ripped it off at 4 a.m. I wrapped yesterday and today when I returned home. All I can say is this binding with three layers of bandages, a layer of cotton and a cotton sleeve underneath is my version of the third ring of hell. When the bandages are removed, there are deep marks into my skin from the compression and that is considered normal. It does reduce the swelling, but there is nothing "normal" about it. At all.

I am confident, however, that my arm will return to normal size and stay that way. It will, it will, it will.

Wednesday, July 7th: Lymphedema Blues

Warning: I'm wallowing in self-pity this week. As promised, I'm keeping it real in documenting my journey, I'm not holding back. I know I'll emerge on the other side of this, but for now I am plowing through a bleak present. I know that this lymphedema will resolve itself and won't be such an overwhelming obstacle soon. Very soon. For now, however, resolution is not on the horizon.

Yesterday my arm swelled up as I was teaching class in the heated room. Helplessly, I watched it blow up over the 75-minute class. It was devastating.

How to analogize: I'd say it is like when you feel the initial tingling of a cold sore popping up at an inopportune time in a conspicuous location. The horror hits you as you realize if you don't catch it in time; it will explode right on the center of your lip, most likely right before you have a big date or photo session. And, you know that it will linger for weeks before it decides to make its exit.

Or, if you haven't had a cold sore, dredge up that buried high school memory when a giant pimple the size of a raspberry sprouted on the tip of your nose before prom.

So, control issues are rearing their ugly heads. When will this be under control? Why another physical issue that forces me to curtail my regular activities? Why so much restriction? Why am I in the 25% to develop this condition? I don't mean to be a big fat baby, but this is making me feel sorry for myself. Period. I'd hoped to focus on regaining my strength and building back up to feeling "normal" again.

Okay, the positive: my new lymphedema therapist is excellent and has some great suggestions and I am praying that they work. Fast. Sleeping with my arm in three layers of bandages and one layer of thick cotton isn't comfortable. In fact, I haven't slept much in four nights. Finally, I ripped them off at 3 a.m. last night.

Okay, manifestation time: I will sleep eight blissful hours tonight and when I wake up in the morning and remove my bandages, my hand will look normal. After I meet with the physical therapist tomorrow, all will be resolved. For the foreseeable future.

Friday, July 9th: Warner Springs-Eve

TGIF! No more appointments for a few days. This week has been dominated by efforts to curb the expansion of my arm. Unfortunately, it is bigger than it was last week, which is not the desired result. So, I'll be wearing a sleeve all day every day and bandages all night for the foreseeable future. Great.

On the alternative front, I'm continuing with the microcurrent treatments that yield immediate results in diminishing swelling. I'm also going to start on some herbal supplements that are supposed to aid with lymphatic system issues. And, I am working my way to true visualization and healing. Lymphedema will resolve and will become a distant memory. No more flare ups. This is it. One-shot evil lymphedema: do your worst! Once you are gone, you are history. Period.

On a positive note, today I met with an amazing woman who works for City of Hope. She is organizing an event called Yoga for Hope to raise money for cancer research. I am going to work with her to help make it a huge success. I'm honored to be a part of this inaugural event.

What is City of Hope? It is one of only 40 National Cancer Institute-designated Comprehensive Cancer Centers nationwide and a founding member of the National Comprehensive Cancer Network. An independent biomedical research, treatment and education institution, it is a leader in the fight to conquer cancer, diabetes, HIV/AIDS and other life-threatening diseases. www.cityofhope.org.

Off to pack for Warner Springs. It is the second annual ActiveX (www.active.com) Endurance Camp at Warner Springs. Arch Fuston organizes a weekend of triathlon preparation, complete with bringing out the experts to coach on tri transitions, swim trials, etc. I'm leading a yoga class on Sunday morning for all the athletes after they return from their run. Last year was a blast and I expect the same for this year.

Sunday, July 11th: A change of scenery

I know there are those who say that you can't run away from your problems, but I tend to disagree. Changing location can play a huge part in altering your mood, at least for a little while. Escape. Respite.
ActiveX Endurance Camp at Warner Springs did it for me, at least until my arm swelled up. But, that is a later rant. About 100 active.com employees spent the weekend biking, swimming and running in preparation for the Solana Beach Triathlon.

We arrived to glorious sunshine yesterday. Hot, sunny blue skies. It felt fantastic. San Diego has been gray, cold and drizzly for over two weeks straight and it weighs on the psyche. We lounged at the pool, soaked up some sun and relaxed. For the first time since the lymphedema developed, I was completely happy. An enjoyable BBQ with a wonderful group of people completed a great day.

Alas, the escape was merely fleeting. I spent yesterday afternoon getting fitted for a sleeve to wear all day, every day, until the lymphedema improves. My physical therapist didn't prescribe a gauntlet/glove for me, just the sleeve. My hand has held a great deal of swelling and from what I've read; you are supposed to have a gauntlet (fingerless) glove to control the hand swelling. What do I know as the patient, right?

I'd gotten over the mental and emotional hurdle and had resolved to wear the damn hideous, uncomfortable, orthopedic stocking-looking thing all day and bandage all night. I want my arm back.

So, yesterday morning, I went to my shift at the cat house at Petco and wore the sleeve. By the end of the two- hour shift, my hand was swollen and red. Not good. I lost it. What am I supposed to do? I'm trying to comply with all of this restrictive treatment and it ISN'T WORKING. I am so frustrated that I cannot stop bursting into tears. Why did my hand swell up? No medical personnel were available to answer my questions.

Then, I bandaged last night after the Warner Springs dinner and expected to wake up to a smaller arm. Nope. No visual difference. It made my morning challenging, trying to ignore it as I taught, worried it would swell more from the efforts.
Escape over.

Tuesday, July 13ᵗʰ: Turning the corner

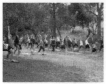

What a difference a day makes. I am so grateful for all the support that I have. Today, I turned the corner in my mindset with this lymphedema. It isn't resolved yet, but I decided that it will be. I am not accepting that this could take six months of daily bandaging and sleeve wearing. I will heal faster because I am strong.

Lois used the microcurrent machine to open up the lymphatic pathways near the incision that represents the inception of this latest snafu in my cancer recuperation. It is miraculous how the swelling subsides so quickly with this alternative treatment. It sure beats bandaging. Anyways, I kissed my arm in the shower and told it that it would be healed very soon. Love, love, love to my right arm.

And, enough about the arm. Way too much airtime over the last three and one-half weeks.

As I mentioned earlier, I was thrilled to go to Warner Springs and participate in active.com's Endurance Camp. Today, I was thrilled to receive feedback from some of the students who practiced yoga with me.

"That was the absolute best yoga experience I've ever had. Period."

"In the top three yoga sessions I've had"

"Claire is amazing. I've been doing this for years, and THAT was amazing."

It makes me all warm and fuzzy inside to know that I can connect with people through my teaching. I love teaching yoga.

Today, things shifted for me. I've closed a chapter and am certain that my strength is returning. My body thinks it is getting poisoned again on Thursday and it isn't! I can't wait to see how I start feeling each day now that my cells aren't under attack from the chemo drugs. And, hair is growing. By next week, I'm sure I'll have a luxurious mane. I can dream big, right?

Wednesday, July 14th: Sunny day number two

San Diego weather is back! Sunny and 75. I wanted to hit the pool, but my arm was bandaged up after therapy and I envisioned a sweaty, messy endeavor. I wouldn't want to scare any of the kids at the pool. Imagine: the bald lady with the big pink hat and Michelin Man arm starts screaming and ripping bandages off, throwing them in the pool. They'd probably be scarred for life.

As the arm shrinks: my arm is smaller than last week, but not as small as the week before. It was 14% larger two weeks ago and *21% larger* last week. Scary. It is down to a 17% difference. My goal is that by my birthday in two weeks...yes, that is right--MY BIRTHDAY IS TWO WEEKS FROM TODAY: JULY 28TH! I MADE IT!!

Okay, my goal is that by my birthday in two weeks, the shrinkage will be under 10%. How many times can I say that my birthday is in two weeks? We are shooting for a 5-10% difference and then maintaining that. Forever. My physical therapist also cleared me to start doing some light weights on my arms and five Sun Salutations. Yippee! I can do five Sun Salutations. On my knees and on my forearms in Down Dog. It is a start.

Tomorrow is a big day. I have physical therapy again at 11:30 a.m. and will be compressed and bandaged when I head over for the CT-Scan from Hell. The Liver Scan. That silly spot is going to be gone, gone, gone. I figured out what it was anyways: remnants from Prom Night.

After the scan, I meet with the radiation oncologist to discuss frying my boob for seven weeks. I am looking forward to tomorrow being over already and I haven't even woken up yet.

Then, a weekend of sunshine! And working out. On the road to recovery. Did I mention that my birthday is in two weeks?

Thursday, July 15th: May I have a redo please?
Today started out fabulously:

7:30 a.m. -- cuddle session with the cats.
8:00 a.m. -- gentle yoga practice at home, all with the Michelin Man arm bandaging.
10:30 a.m. -- manicure/pedicure. That's when it headed south.

My Fantasy Day: I would've gone to see *Eclipse* again by myself. Next, I would read my new book as I basked in the sun at the pool. Since this is my fantasy, I would play with the cats and then walk on the beach with my man.
My Actual Day: 11:30 a.m. -- Lymphedema therapy, complete with compression pump and bandaging.

1:10 p.m. -- Check in at Radiology for the re-scan of the liver. No pressure or stress there. Drank a pitcher of dye slowly for an hour and a quarter, had an IV inserted into my arm which contained more dye and then was stuffed into the Scanner. You may recall me discussing that fun test where they inject dye through the IV and it instantly makes you feel like you wet your pants. Silver lining: graham crackers and orange juice if you make it out without requiring a diaper.

3:35 p.m. -- Famished after fasting all morning for liver scan. Go to Green Hospital cafeteria. Go directly to baked goods bin. Purchase two cookies and a jelly donut. Inhale in less than two minutes. Not much chewing. Twenty minutes later, for some odd reason, I developed an intense tummy ache. I guess that wasn't the super-antioxidant meal I should've had. Oh well.

4:00 p.m. -- Report to Radiation Oncology in basement of Scripps Clinic. Receive my nifty removable armband that will enable me to park for free for the next seven and one-half weeks of daily radiation treatment. I've always loved VIP treatment.

The nurse weighs me and I weigh more than I ever have in my entire LIFE. Are you kidding me? So, on top of everything I am fat. Those cookies sure registered quickly. Then, I get the scoop: the doctor isn't going to radiate my lymph nodes because that will make the lymphedema worse. And, he informs me that since the cancer in my one lymph node had only been 4mm, read TINY, that he felt comfortable radiating just my breast.

How can I not feel devastated to discover that tiny 4mm spot was the difference between the axial dissection that required chemo and caused lymphedema and having the lesser invasive lumpectomy and radiation? 4 mm was the game changer. No chemo. No baldness. No lymphedema.

Nobody can explain to me why I have to have radiation after having had chemo. Chemo was supposed to kill every microscopic cell, cancer or not, right? Isn't this a bit much to now radiate my breast 36 times?

The day wasn't over yet: they mark up the area where they plan on radiating you. With magic markers and stickers. I felt like a prize cantaloupe at the county fair.

Then, you put your arms overhead and get shoveled into yet another CT scanner while they photograph the exact location for treatment. They also take photos with a regular camera. What the heck am I going to do when I get famous and those are leaked on the Internet?

Next, they remove the stickers and permanently tattoo you in three different spots. Mind you, I was not of the generation who felt compelled to get a tattoo. No desire. Ever. Now, I have a dot right in the middle of my cleavage. Great. Couldn't they do it on the boob where it could be covered up? And, the tech was really sweet and attempted to make the spot tiny. This kindness backfired and she had to re-poke me with the needle in two of three spots. It hurt. A lot.

I prefer Scenario One: my fantasy day. Thank you very much.

Saturday, July 17th: A normal summer night

It feels like summer! Normal summer, not Ye Olde Summer of Cancer 2010. Wonderful. Dinner in Laguna last night was lovely. What a gorgeous little seaside town. I did whip off Sheila the second we got into the car and rode back to Carlsbad bald. Not so normal!

Today, I had nothing to do, nowhere to be. I'd almost forgotten how that feels. We headed down to the beach and basked in the sun and splashed in the surf. I sported

Dominique with a straw hat. I only went into the ocean up to my thighs because Dominique can't swim!

We reviewed our Australia travel book and the trip is beginning to take shape. Reality! Escape! Two weeks of bliss! Two months from today we are on the plane to Sydney.

This morning, I unwrapped my bandaged arm and was thrilled to see my hand looking smaller than it has in the last few weeks. Almost normal. Veins and tendons and wrinkles and everything. It maintained all day! I did some yoga here at the house, but re-bandaged it first. I'm not taking any chances! Perhaps I've broken the barrier and the miracle has arrived: no more swelling.

People have been asking how I am feeling. Well, my body feels bizarre. My energy level feels like it is increasing. No more mandatory naps. But, my legs are incredibly sore, as if I'd climbed El Capitan. Stop laughing at that visual. I also feel swollen all over. Perhaps the lactic acid is reacting differently? I'm not sure what causes these quick shifts in my physique. Maybe every cell in my body is dancing because they've realized the chemotherapy portion of treatment is done, done, done. That's great and all, but they can rein it in a bit because my pants feel tight.

I've been pondering the next two months of daily radiation and I am not convinced, at all, that it is the right thing to do. Why can't the doctors give me recurrence numbers specifically for 1) surgery + 2) chemotherapy + 3) radiation??? They keep saying that lumpectomy goes with radiation, whether or not lymph nodes are involved. But, they've told me that the chemotherapy kills everything. Why do I need to cook my right boob and surrounding environs? What damage will that do to my skin, my muscle, my bone, and my organs?

Tuesday, July 27th: Birthday-eve

Do you know those days where you are running from place to place, always about five minutes late for each appointment? I had one of those frenetic days today for the first time that I can recall. Hectic schedules used to be a mainstay and I must say that I do not miss the madness.

I won't bore you with all the details, but I must rant about my ridiculous morning at Scripps. I reported to Radiation Oncology at 9 a.m. for my radiation and repeat CT-Scan. Yes, repeat CT-Scan.

Apparently, the one that was taken the day I was tattooed turned out strangely. Two techs asked me if I'd been panting during the scan. Panting. My bafflement must have shown because one lady actually panted like a dog to illustrate. I assured all of them that I hadn't been laying there, in all of my magic marker and stickered glory, panting.

Anyways, they told me to expect to be there for an hour. My lymphedema physical therapy appointment was at 10 a.m. at the Scripps La Jolla location, about five minutes away. I could make that work. After the CT-Scan, however, the story changes and they tell me that it will be at least an hour before they'd have things set up for radiation. And, that I'd need to redo the X-rays from the day before because the parameters were all wrong from the CT-scan where I was allegedly panting. Well, what the heck did they radiate yesterday then? If all the X-rays and CT-scan were wrong and needed redoing, should I be concerned?

Beyond concern, I was annoyed. They asked if I could come back, assuring me that they'd have me out of there in 10-15 minutes. I told them no, that I had an appointment at 10 a.m., class at noon, and appointments at 2, 3:30 and 4:30 p.m. I'd come for my allotted hour and that wasn't enough?

Persistent creatures that they are, they asked if I could return for 10 to 15 minutes after my 10 a.m. physical therapy appointment and assured me I'd be able to make it to Encinitas for my noon class. So, I zoom over to Scripps La Jolla for physical therapy. I cut my appointment 30 minutes short. Mind you, this is the second robe I've changed into by 10 a.m.

I then run from physical therapy, hop in my car and careen back over to the parking lot from hell at Scripps Torrey Pines. For the second time, I battled octogenarians (sorry Dad) who felt free to drive the wrong way up one-way lanes, lay on the horn while reversing up said lane in attempts to snag parking spaces. Madness. They need to sell extra insurance to traverse that lot.

I park. I gallop back into the basement to Radiation. On goes Robe Number Three, accidentally ripping off Sheila in the process. I plopped her back on my head, slightly askew, in my haste to get my radiation. Tick tock. Fifteen minutes elapse in the waiting area. It is now 11:33 and I need to be in Encinitas in half an hour. My agreement with these people was that I'd run back to them and they'd get me in and out in 15 minutes. My blood was boiling at this point.

No-showing my class wasn't an option, so I trotted back to shed Robe Number Three and hightailed out. I let the receptionist know that I had to leave and that I wasn't returning a third time. I had to run back up the stairs, risk my life navigating the parking lot, and speed all the way to Encinitas and then try to calm myself down enough to teach class.

Wow, this is the non-detailed version. The day improved from there.

I'm really excited for tomorrow's trip to Laguna with Todd. It will start with an 8:30 a.m. radiation appointment. After that, it is celebration time!

Thursday, July 29th: Birthday escape recap

My birthday was fantastic! Thank you everyone for all the birthday cards and wishes!

My primary desire was for sunshine and an escape from the reality of continued treatment. After an 8:30 a.m. radiation session, where anyone and everyone profusely apologized to me for Tuesday, Todd and I zoomed up to Laguna Beach for a 26-hour escape. I highly recommend the Casa Laguna Inn Bed & Breakfast for a perfect trip that made us feel like we were on the French Riviera.

With the sun shining brightly, the sky a clear blue and the air warm and soft, we headed north. I was so excited to leave my radiation treatment behind that I didn't mind wearing my Solaris arm-length oven-mitt in the car. I knew that I was not wearing the sleeve for most of the day and figured that would compensate. We headed to Splashes for lunch. Splashes is the restaurant at the fancy Surf & Sand Resort. We dined with the ladies who lunch. Rather decadent for a Wednesday afternoon.

Then, we meandered down to our B&B. It was built circa 1920 and is filled with terraces and courtyards and winding vines tipped with bougainvillea. We lounged by the pool with a breathtaking view of the ocean, where classical music softly played in the background. It felt so healing to bask in the sun, with the occasional dip in the pool. Next, we checked into our room, which was on the top level, with a view of the Pacific I could get accustomed to. We rounded out the afternoon with a walk down to Victoria Beach and some wine and cheese from the B&B happy hour.

Laguna has a free shuttle trolley that transported us a few miles into the center of town. We enjoyed dinner at Hush, a rather modern California cuisine restaurant. Another exquisite meal. Enjoying food is such an important part of living in the present moment. I'm so glad that my taste buds are returning to normal. Now, I have to admit that we drank a lot of wine and I'm a lightweight. Let's just say that I'm happy my exit from the trolley in four-inch heels was not captured on film.

After enjoying a tasty breakfast on the terrace, strolling around town and hitting the beach, we returned to San Diego. And, the birthday buzz screamed to a halt as I headed down to Scripps for my radiation treatment.

My take on radiation thus far: the treatment is fast and they run it like clockwork. But, I'm concerned that I already feel the heat and tightness in my skin. Wow, what will it be like come September? I'm slathering on the aloe and plan on purchasing some calendula cream because it is supposed to be good at preventing the serious skin damage that can occur. My poor boob has just endured some serious abuse this year. I cannot wait for September 15th: the last day of radiation, and just two days before we leave for Australia. Talk about a welcome escape!

Saturday, July 31st: Yoga for cancer recovery series

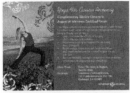

Let's talk about silver linings: my original theme for this blogging endeavor. Please take a look at the invitation above and I think you'll see one of the primary gifts I've received this year.

While I was going through chemotherapy, I earned my certification to teach yoga to cancer patients. Now that I'm approaching the treatment finish line, I'm able to share what I've learned both on and off of the mat with others who are living with cancer. I am both excited and nervous for the first official series of classes that I'll be teaching in this niche. It is funny: I'm so comfortable teaching yoga; it is as natural to me as breathing.

But this is different. More powerful because there is an additional bond between all of the students that automatically makes us kindred souls: our lives have been touched in a way that changes us forever. So, I'm nervous. I want to share my gift of teaching with this community, to help heal, to help make a difference. I want to resonate.

I'm excited to be partnering with lululemon Carlsbad, where I am an ambassador, in offering this series of free weekly classes for the month of August. We'll meet Thursday mornings at 9 a.m., prior to the store opening, starting next week. The classes are open to all levels and all people living with cancer; the only requirement is showing up on the mat.

Chapter 8: August

August 1st: Best Ladies in LA

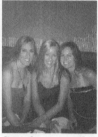

Sunday evenings always seem to be a time for reflection for me.

I just returned from a quick trip to La-la land to visit Joanna and Angie to celebrate all three of our birthdays. As always, it was wonderful to catch up and hang out with two of my best friends! I made them both try on my Solaris night sleeve so they could get a feel for my new sleeping attire. I also made them go for a walk with me in my orthopedic stocking-looking sleeve and fingerless glove. In Beverly Hills, no less. That's what friends are for, right?

Actually, I had lots of time to reflect while driving up and back. Sadly, I was not kissed by the karma fairy in the traffic department. It was nasty bumper to bumper both ways. Between the bouts of mind-numbing brake riding and careening 80 miles an hour down the highway, I managed to process some thoughts that have been circling around in my brain.

With about half of my classes on hold for the foreseeable future, I've got more time and less money. Inverse of what one would usually seek. Part of me had the knee-jerk reaction to reach out and call studios and pick up classes elsewhere pronto! Work, work, work. But listening to my gut, I know this isn't the right thing to do. I am starting the Yoga for Cancer Recovery at lululemon and will be teaching it weekly for August. I want these classes to be really special and that is a primary focus.

My dance card is rather full with daily radiation field trips consuming roughly two hours altogether, including driving time. Ten hours a week: a part-time job! And, another few hours working with my acupuncturist to free up the lymph node blockage. Five to seven lymphatic self-massages a day: another 45 minutes. No wonder the thought of beginning new classes seems formidable.

Epiphany: I need to just chill out and teach my current classes until radiation ends. People keep telling me that I'll be exhausted the last few weeks of treatment. I already feel a weird wave of nausea/tiredness each time I've stepped off the radiation table. But I'm taking a whole slew of new, very expensive supplements, designed to help me rebuild my immune system and battle these side effects. I'm getting tired just thinking about it.

I'm supposed to start my first coaching class tomorrow. And, I don't feel particularly enthusiastic, which worries me. Usually, I am the big dork with sharpened pencils, new notebooks and fresh highlighters, ready to absorb new information. Especially because I believe that the coaching education will be invaluable for me in my quest to help others down the line. But I'm just not feeling it right now. How can I do well if I'm not excited? I am notorious for acing any class that interests me and just not caring about the others. I'm seriously considering calling CoachU tomorrow and postponing everything until early 2011. My mind and heart don't feel engaged.

I really just feel like focusing on teaching yoga, developing a cool program for Yoga for Cancer Recovery above and beyond the August series, working with City of Hope planning the landmark event Yoga for Hope and writing. I'm feeling the pull to dig out my half-finished romance novel, yes, romance novel, and completing it. It is set in Laguna Beach and I've got Laguna fresh on my mind after our wonderful trip there last week. Azure ocean, emerald green trees and bougainvillea to spare.

We'll see what Monday brings.

Monday, August 2nd: Ovation Cell Therapy!

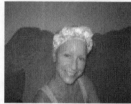

Not much to say when the photo says it all.

Ovation Cell Therapy! Grow hair, grow! So, you slather on the coconut-smelling concoction all over your scalp and leave it on for a few hours. I utilized the shower cap that I swiped from the Laguna B&B last week. For everyone who has asked how Todd is handling all of this: this is the Claire that he gets to enjoy behind closed doors. No wig, barely any eyebrows and a shower cap over my big bald head. Ahhhh, the romance, the beauty, the reality.

I swear that several hundred more little hairs sprouted after I rinsed off my head. I can't wait to have a full, shiny head of hair again. Grow, grow, *grow!!*

Tuesday, August 3rd: Affirmations

Everything you say is an affirmation. Everything you think is an affirmation. Everything! What you want to do is to get control of what you are saying and thinking, so these things bring you good experiences in life rather than rotten experiences. Louise Hay

I love this quote from Louise Hay. Come to think of it, I love several quotes from Louise Hay: brilliant woman. With what I've been experiencing this year, I'm finding it increasingly important to make sure that I'm very careful where I allow my thoughts to wander. If I am not disciplined, I can spiral downward at an alarming rate.

An example? The swelling in my hand from the lymphedema can completely freak me out in a flash. When it was really bad a few weeks ago, I was convinced that I would be completely disabled with my writing hand, never write again, never wear a ring, and never want to talk with my hands again. Mind you, my father has joked that if my hands were tied behind my back, I would be rendered mute because I tend to gesture so wildly to emphasize a point. Not an exaggeration.

A multitude of factors conspired to drag me out of a positive mindset: the isolation in not being able to do a lot of my favorite things with my favorite people. The isolation in not feeling like leaving the house because it is too much effort to pencil on eyebrows and select a wig or hat. The isolation in avoiding talking to people because I am a broken record stuck on the damn arm or radiation or growing hair or something cancer-related.

This morning was a rough one. I didn't sleep at all last night between the night sleeve pinching me and Oreo howling all evening. Methinks he needs his steroid shot because he is obviously not feeling well. That is another story.

Being sleep deprived tends to depress me. All I wanted to do was hole up in my house. I went so far as half-heartedly trying to find a sub for my noon yoga class. Luckily, I did go teach and once again, the Frogs yogis were responsible for lifting my mood. It is truly amazing what all of that positive energy does for me. Is that selfish? I can only hope that it is truly reciprocal.

In the spirit of Louise Hay: I will be diligent in choosing my affirmations. I will sleep peacefully for at least eight straight hours tonight. I will have lovely dreams. I will awake tomorrow feeling refreshed and happy.

Thursday, August 5th: Riding the waves

Fluctuations dominate my days. One minute, I feel calm, peaceful and centered and the next moment melancholy descends. I guess the good news is that these shifts are fleeting and I am confident that they will pass.

On a positive note, the first Yoga for Cancer Recovery class at lululemon was a success this morning. I was lucky enough to have a fellow teacher, Irina, assist me. Seven students came and I am hopeful that they enjoyed the class as much as I enjoyed teaching it. Patti, my wonderful wig lady, came and loved it! I'm so thrilled that I could give back to her. I can't wait for next week, same bat time, same bat channel. I also learned that there is another class offered at the Cancer Center in Encinitas on Tuesday morning, so I am going to partake of that one next week.

On a less positive note, once a week, I get weighed and meet with the doctor to check in on how I am feeling. I don't understand why they weigh me? Are they afraid they might fry too many pounds off of me? As I drove through McDonald's, yes McDonald's, this afternoon, I don't think there is any danger of me wasting away. I've been doing a lot of emotional eating this week: goes with the oscillation I suppose! The good news is that I could taste the salt on the McDonald's French fries. Hallelujah! The taste buds are back!

I digress. I had an interesting conversation with my Radiation Oncologist this afternoon. When he asked me how my energy levels were, I replied that they were great, probably because of all the supplements I'm taking. Well, he and the nurse jumped on the supplement soapbox. They informed me that I could take a multivitamin, but not take any antioxidants. Apparently, radiation is oxidizing and the antioxidants could prevent it from working. Really. Seriously, I cannot fathom how the death rays could be thwarted by some antioxidants.

Wouldn't that be like me trying to fight off an armored tank with a slingshot? I don't buy it and I am going to continue to take them.

Actually, my energy level is most likely attributable to the acupuncture that I've been receiving. And, it is only the second week of radiation. I understand that it is cumulative and I've got five and one-half weeks to go.

What may kill me is the parking lot at Scripps. It is a perilous lot, with at least half the drivers too blind to see, too drugged up to drive or too upset to navigate. I swear if "Seinfeld" were still on the air, the Scripps parking lot would serve as fodder for at least a week of episodes. I need a chauffeur! But I better make sure I'm dropped off right at the curb or one of the aforementioned vehicles will run me down.

Friday, August 6th: Back to the Jeannie bottle

I want to hop into my cozy 'I Dream of Jeannie" bottle and not emerge until September 16th. Why the 16th? Radiation ends the 15th and we leave for Australia on the 17th. That will give me a day to pack and prepare for the trip.

I'm feeling psychologically exhausted right now. My physical energy is fine, but this mental and emotional battle I've been waging all year is sapping my strength. At times, I am silent yet screaming in my head. I wonder if people can tell? The final straw, yes there seems to be a final straw collection, is that last night I realized that I'd lost most of my eyebrows and at least three-quarters of my precious eyelashes.

Before you say, 'But you are alive,' yes, I know that I'm alive. And, I am grateful. Truly, I am grateful for my wonderful boyfriend, friends and family. But unless you've endured this treatment and lived with so many crappy side effects, you cannot understand how upsetting it is when these very visible symbols that you are sick keep slapping you in the face. Kind of like the hot flash that is drenching the back of my tank top as I write this.

I'm like a Monet painting: look great from far away and then you focus and notice that the eyebrows are painted on like the Fairfax Hospital cafeteria lady, that there are about 10 eyelashes total between both eyes, that the hair is a wig and that there is an ugly beige sleeve and glove on my right arm and hand. And, possible sweat stains from a hot flash.

Mind you, it took 10 minutes to create said eyebrows and individually apply mascara to the sparse, long spindly lashes. How did they fall out six weeks after chemotherapy? I committed the grave error of going online to research this distressing issue and instead of finding an answer found some information that Taxotere, one of the chemo drugs I was fed, can cause permanent hair loss. Fantastic news.

Let's see, on a positive note: my arm looks the best today than it has in the seven weeks that I've been dealing with this lymphedema. Perhaps it is finally going to stabilize and allow me to continue increasing my exercise and walk around bare-armed.

So, Jeannie bottle, here I come. I'm tired of this daily battle and just want to go to sleep and wake up next month. Hopefully with some lashes, brows and hair.

Saturday, August 7th: But I'm alive, right?

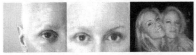

I cannot sleep. Nothing new.

Here are two photos of me this morning and one of me pre-cancer. I know that these eyelashes and brows will come back one day, but this really stinks. One photo is the eye and eyebrow sans makeup. Notice the lovely bald head. The second shot shows me after I spent 10 minutes drawing on brows and carefully crafting eye-makeup on one side. The pre-cancer shot with my friend Nikki shows me with eyebrows and my beautiful long lashes that I got courtesy of my dear papa.

They say eyes are the windows of the soul. My eyes now finally reveal my illness to anyone and everyone. They scream that I am sick. Constantly red-rimmed, constantly puffy, no lashes, no brows. Nowhere to hide. Hideous.

Doctors, nurses, everyone really keeps telling me the same thing: 'Be grateful that you're alive!' You are so young, all this is temporary, and you'll live a long healthy life if you do as we say. Chemotherapy will destroy your ovaries and you'll be in early menopause, but you're alive! You'll lose your hair, your brows and lashes, you'll have scars and tattoos for a lifetime, but you're alive! You may get lymphedema and have to sleep in bandages or an incredibly tight compression sleeve for the rest of your life, but you're alive! Who the hell knows what this daily radiation will do to you, but suck it up because you are alive! Take Tamoxifin for the next five years or else your odds of being alive sharply decline!

Back when this all began unfolding in its terrible, surreal way, I didn't want all of these drugs. Of course I want to live, but at what cost?

The irony is that they can't even tell me if I am cancer-free. Isn't that crazy? There are no guarantees and I am not certain that I've made the right choices jumping on this surgery-chemo-radiation assembly line. Back to that basic discussion of quality vs. quantity. The Short Happy Life of Claire Petretti or The Long Sick Half-Life?

I've had the lyrics of Pearl Jam's "Alive" in my head for a while now. Today the volume increased and I cannot ignore it nor turn off the music.

"Alive" by Pearl Jam, excerpt:
I, I'm still alive
Hey I, but, I'm still alive
Hey I, boy, I'm still alive
Hey I, I, I, I'm still alive, yeah
Ooh yeah...yeah yeah yeah...oh...oh...
"Is something wrong?" she said
Of course there is

"You're still alive," she said
Oh, and do I deserve to be?
Is that the question?
And if so...if so...who answers...who answers...?
I, oh, I'm still alive
Hey I, oh, I'm still alive
Hey I, but, I'm still alive
Yeah I, ooh, I'm still alive
Yeah yeah yeah yeah yeah yeah

Sunday, August 8th: Sunshine works its magic

And, the rollercoaster ascends again. Not a moment too soon.

Kirsten and I met in Cardiff for a morning beach walk. The sun was shining, the ocean was a clear and stunning blue and it felt fabulous to be outside. The Cardiff beach walk used to be an at least bi-weekly ritual and it felt great to return to it. I've missed this type of time spent with my friends.

My legs are feeling stronger and each day I'm walking farther. I'm thrilled! Yesterday Todd and I walked the whole lagoon for the first time in several months. And, my arm has been holding steady since Friday. Perhaps I've turned a corner with the lymphedema.

Now, it is time to check if any more hair has sprouted.

Tuesday, August 10th: Holding steady

Paring down my schedule and adding in more daily exercise seems to be doing the trick. I'm feeling more balanced and a little less out of control. I'm so thrilled that I've been able to walk about an hour a day. I've missed it so much. Now that my legs don't feel like I hiked Everest, I feel freer.

223

Even more exciting is that my arm continues to hold steady at just about normal size. Who knew how thrilling it would be to see my pointy elbow again? I'm continuing to add more activity for my upper body. In fact, at this rate I'll be a veritable Wonder Woman: I've built up to two sets of various exercises with three-pound weights. Pretty funny. But it is a start. I'm so grateful that I'm able to do something without the fear of my forearm and hand blowing up like a balloon.

Slowly.

McCabe, my artist friend, came over to see if she could spice up my orthopedic beige sleeve. I was considering making it look like I have a full-sleeve tattoo on that arm! It could be fun for yoga! I plan on weaning off of the sleeve as soon as I can, but will wear it to workout for the foreseeable future: better safe than sorry. I would probably go batty if I had to endure another seven-and-one-half-week blow-up again. Also, I know that I pooh-poohed *www.lymphedivas.com* in the past, but they have tons of cool styles, like diamond trim. I stand corrected.

McCabe is also a scarf expert, yet another area where I am not gifted, and brought me a gorgeous scarf to wear with the hat hair. She tied it too. I'm hoping that I can just slip it on already tied because otherwise I might be in trouble. We are digging deep to find my inner bohemian chic. Very deep. I'm half-French for goodness sakes! You'd think I'd be gifted with scarves. Or chic.

Week three of radiation is in full swing and it shows. My skin is pink with small red polka-dots. Lovely. I'm slathering on calendula lotion at least four times a day to help counteract the radiation, but methinks the large beam will win. So, although I've got three fabulous new bikinis,

I now need to cover up the top and make sure I don't get sun.

I can't believe that it is almost the middle of August. I wonder how I will feel next August when I reflect back upon 2010? At the moment, I don't have a clue. I've survived a lot of loss and ups and downs in my life, but making it through to the other side of this journey will definitely leave me a changed woman. Mind, body, spirit. I am truly grateful for everyone in my life: I'm blessed to have so much support and love surrounding me through this rollercoaster ride.

Thursday, August 12th: City of Hope tour

Yesterday, I was lucky enough to be part of a tour of the City of Hope in Duarte, California. In March, I'll be chairing the inaugural Yoga for Hope in San Diego.

Their motto: **There is no profit in curing the body if in the process we destroy the soul.**

This really struck me because if anything can steal your soul and crush your essence, it is walking this walk. If only all cancer-treatment centers operated the same way. City of Hope is truly a unique research and treatment facility.

They are pioneers in cutting-edge research for cancer, HIV and diabetes. This trio of diseases is extremely personal to me and I've been very emotional since actually setting foot on the 120-acre City yesterday.

The cancer is personal to me and to my sister who is a five-year survivor (go Yael!).

The diabetes is personal to me as my oldest and best friend is a Type 1 diabetic.

The HIV is personal to me because I lost my brothers Paul and Andre to the disease. Paul was 27 years old when he passed; Andre was 33.

Today, I am truly feeling weighed down by all of these challenges and by all of the loss. I miss my brothers. I've got another four and one-half weeks of daily radiation and I just wish I could go to sleep and wake up and it would be over. I'd also like to wake up with my eyelashes returned to me. Every single long, black one of them.

I did squeeze in a lovely walk on the beach at Torrey Pines after acupuncture, prior to radiation. I could feel the healing ocean breeze caressing my skin, giving me strength to continue on with my treatment. It feels good to know that all I have to do over the next three days is teach class in the morning, get radiation, volunteer with the cats Saturday morning and that is it. Weekend time!

Saturday, August 14th: Hot Flashes!

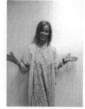

I'm having a hot flash. Not exactly how I envisioned spending my Saturday night. It begins with the back of my neck beginning to cook. Literally. The heat then spreads down my back and creates a lovely film of sweat designed to make whatever I'm wearing stick to my back. You know, like when you are in Washington, D.C. on any given summer day and leave your air-conditioned house and step into the 90% humidity and are instantly drenched? No need for travel: I get to sweat in the comfort of my own home.

Hot flashes are yet another one of those side effects that is downplayed. Like losing your hair. The doctor casually relays a laundry list of potential side effects like, "You'll have some hot flashes and may go into menopause about 10 years early." Or, "Your underarm? That will be numb forever, didn't we mention that?" "Lymphedema, you can never go in a hot tub or sauna again and definitely don't lift more than 15 pounds. You make your living teaching yoga in a heated room? Time for a career change." I could continue.

This photo shows my daily attire for radiation treatment. Please note my lovely sleeve and glove. For radiation, each day I walk back to the dressing room, lock the door and change into two robes. About one-third of the time I end up accidentally yanking off my hair of the day in the process.

Speaking of wigs, you may notice that I am sporting a new look in said photo. The brilliant and incomparable Patti Joyce has created another masterpiece. I told her that I was close to throwing Sheila out the window of my car because the heat makes her stick to the back of my neck. In an effort to prevent a pile-up on the highway, Patti found one just like Sheila, but shorter. And, voila: here it is! I haven't named her yet. But she is lighter, pretty cute and should get me through until my hair is long enough to go wigless. (The photo is kind of dark--it is the same Pralines-'n-Cream color as Sheila)

The lovely Lori was kind enough to take me to radiation because she was worried I might lose my last marble in the dreaded Scripps parking lot. Of course, there were plenty of open spots when she drove me. Not a crazy lunatic to be seen. No 90 year olds honking and reversing across the lot at 60 mph. No back-up out onto Torrey

Pines Road. It figures. I swear the parking lot is usually a nightmare.

Fourteen Radiations down. Twenty-two to go. Less than five weeks to Australia.

Hang on Petretti. Don't lose your mind when you are so close to the finish line...

Monday, August 16*th*: A thread...

"Anyone can give up; it's the easiest thing in the world to do. But to hold it together when everyone else would understand if you fell apart, that's true strength." - author unknown

What an awesome quote at an auspicious time. My daily Morning Mantra emails are so often right on point. I'm struggling to hold it together. This weekend was an emotional rollercoaster. At this point, I'm scraping the bottom of the energy jar.

I cannot resist the desire to sleep and not awake until a few days before we head to Australia. Or, should I say, I'd like time to freeze because I don't want to miss any of the many positive things I've got going on over the next month.

I guess therein lies my answer, right? If I withdraw, I'll miss so much amazing living: teaching, spending time with Todd and my friends, planning Yoga for Hope, attending Taste of Hope this weekend, watching my hair, eyelashes and eyebrows grow back and living a life with gratitude. Nonetheless, checking out seems the most attractive option.

Tuesday, August 17th: Rolling back up

Today was an absolutely beautiful day. Although I had to fork over $1,252.00 to have three mysterious items repaired on my car, something about sensors and thermostats and valves, I didn't freak out. Bonus: this expensive repair job came with a complimentary car wash and rim polish.

As seems to be the pattern, the rollercoaster ascends again. I'm getting whiplash from all of the ups and downs on this ride. I suppose it makes sense that some days are just totally black and depressing and seemingly hopeless. The extremity of the dips and crests continue to surprise me.

The sun rose early this morning: a perfect summer morning. Such a relief after the heavy marine layer that has rendered San Diego a perfect movie set for *Wuthering Heights* or *Pride and Prejudice*. Over the gloomy weekend, I'd expected Heathcliff to come galloping out of the fog. Depressing.

Today, I met with a new private yoga client. She is a breast cancer survivor who wanted to start yoga to recuperate from the prior year of treatment. We had a great session and I think we will work really well together. I'm excited at the direction my career is taking. Ironic that it took cancer to assist me in finding this niche. Don't get me wrong: I love teaching my Power Yoga classes and will continue to do so, but there is a deep satisfaction in making a difference with other survivors by sharing my passion.

Todd and I went for a long walk on the beach. It is so beautiful: I feel so lucky that I actually get to live here!

Clear gorgeous ocean, long stretches of golden sand and cool breezes. Perfect.

And, I wore the smaller-sized sleeve that I couldn't get on two months ago because my arm was so FAT. Yippee! I'm approaching two weeks with a semi-normal-sized arm and am ready to wean slowly off the sleeve and to step up the workouts. I'm beginning to feel like I'm in my own body again. Finally.

In terms of the radiation side effects, my skin is really starting to pinken. The wise Lizzy advised me to use Emu oil and I ran out and snapped some up at Henry's. I used it right after my radiation roasting this afternoon. Between that and the calendula lotion, I hope that my skin doesn't continue to deteriorate.

The end is in sight: September 15th. Countdown to Oz.

Thursday, August 19th: A very good day

Today was fabulous. It was another reminder that even though I've had black moments, by traversing through them I continue to discover happiness again. Faith and hope.

This morning I taught my third of four Yoga for Cancer Recovery classes at lululemon in Carlsbad. We had the biggest class yet with some "regulars" and some new faces. It went great and the feedback continues to be positive. I love it! I met Angela, who is the co-founder of the Young Survival Coalition in San Diego, a group for young women dealing with cancer (www.youngsurvival.org/sandiego). I'd like to get more involved with them.

I'm also trying to figure out the best studio for holding ongoing classes when this series concludes next week. I'd like to offer weekly Yoga for Cancer Recovery classes on a donation basis in North County. Very soon!

The sun continues to shine on San Diego and with each sunny day, my mood shifts a little higher. Radiation, no problem. Check-up with oncologist, piece of cake. Walk on the beach and a few margaritas with Lissa, fabulous!

I was thrilled to return home and find my Lymphedivas package. The two new sleeves are totally cute: much more attractive than the beige. Unfortunately, they sent me the wrong-sized gauntlet and I cannot wear the sleeve without the gauntlet. Waah! I want to wear my new sleeve to teach tomorrow. How funny is it to look back at how I wouldn't even look at the Lymphedivas Web site and now I'm upset that I can't wear my new sleeve soon enough. Interesting how things shift...And, tomorrow is Friday!

Saturday, August 21st: Appropriate beach attire...

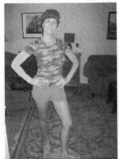

Ahhh, the daily dilemma was actually quite amusing. What the heck was I going to wear to cover my salt-and-pepper chia-pet head and radiation-burned chest to bike to the beach via my new beach cruiser? The weather is pristine and there is no way I was missing out on the beach with Todd today. It was going to be a high-maintenance endeavor.

The issues:

1. Chest must be covered completely because of nasty radiation rash.
2. Need to wear lymphedema sleeve to ride bicycle and walk on beach
3. Need to wear something to cover the head that wouldn't blow off as I cruised down the hill toward the beach. The wigs and hat hair just weren't viable. We have to cross the 5 Freeway and I could just visualize my wig or hat hair flying off into oncoming traffic. Is it a bird? A plane? Or Britney or Gisele? Who cares because it caused a multi-car pileup?

For the bosom, first I tried the rash guard. It is totally cute, but it made me sweat in the house so not an option for the beach. No. Next, I dug out my Corepower Yoga boot camp T-shirt and that was a Yes. Unfortunately, CLAIRE is plastered on the back of it in neon yellow, so everyone from our house to the beach knows that the crazy bicycling bald lady with the weird arm is named CLAIRE.

For the big bald noggin, I layered Todd's buff underneath my favorite baseball cap. If the hat blew off on the bicycle ride, I'd at least be covered.

The arm was just going to look like a prosthetic with the ugly beige with glove.

It worked! See the complete ensemble pictured above. Anyone who has EVER commented on my ego: take note! I felt so liberated and happy cruising on the bicycle and walking on the beach with Todd. Cancer be damned. And, honestly, who would recognize me in that get-up? Repercussions: sweating like a filthy animal on the return uphill bike ride. My head was drenched with sweat, as was the rest of me. But, it was worth it!

To maintain my great mood, I'm not going to compare these photos to the bikini shots from the past. But, I was just as happy to be out on the beach today as I was then.

Sunday, August 22nd: Grow baby grow!

Today is the first day of a three-day weekend with nothing really scheduled: lovely and relaxing. And, it appears that the sun is actually going to show through the heavy marine layer that has been cloaking San Diego since Thursday. Come on sun!

I can't wait for my radiated red skin to heal! The skin under my arm has now blistered, broken up, and rubbed raw a few times. No matter how much ointment I slather on it, the location just sucks. And, to reminisce that the doctor told me that antioxidants might prevent the radiation from working? I had the last radiation to that area on Thursday and the final seven are just to the lumpectomy incision. I'm optimistic that the rest of the area will be healed by next week.

Todd and I are leaving for Australia in less than two weeks! I cannot believe it. The days are taking shape and so is my vacation wardrobe. I've lucked out with finding some shorts and walking shoes and a few other fun things that scream vacation time! Sydney! Melbourne! Great Ocean Road!

I am willing my hair to grow fast enough that Sheila, Sydney, Britney and Gisele are shadows of my past! I'd love to go to Australia with a bare head and not worry about wigs. In that spirit, I've got Ovation slathered on my head with the shower cap on top. Pretty.

If you missed that photo from a few weeks ago, scroll back to see it. I look the same, but now I have my own eyebrows and eyelashes. A lot of eyebrows. It is amazing how fast the brow hair is growing! At this rate, I will resemble Brooke Shields circa the 1980s. I've got an appointment with my hairdresser on the 16th, the day before we leave, to put some color on this head. I have no problem sporting a crew cut, but not a predominantly silver one. No way. No how.

I'm so happy to be approaching the conclusion of this ride. I found the lump on January 2nd and treatment is finished on September 15th. The light at the end of the tunnel brightens by the hour.

Tuesday, August 24th: Feeling grateful

I've been feeling very grateful for all of the blessings in my life these days. One of the primary "silver linings" in this cancer ride comes in the form of the numerous amazing people that I've met or reconnected with since January. My friends have been incredible: consistently supportive, kind, and caring. I am so lucky to be buoyed up by all the positive energy.

And, I see the light at the end of the tunnel! As I cross off each day of radiation with my red pen, I feel lighter. Twenty-one down, 15 to go. My skin looks wretched. Despite a heavy slathering of Aquaphor, it is itchy and incredibly annoying. Nonetheless, burned, rash-covered flesh in an isolated area of the body still beats chemo side effects.

Speaking of chemo side effects: hair is sprouting at an incredible rate! Everywhere. Who would have believed that I would need a bikini wax before I needed an eyebrow wax? Believe it.

234

Todd rubs my fuzzy head, singing 'Chia, Chia, Chia.' I don't mind, even though it is silver and brown. My eyebrows are a rather strange charcoal color: again, better than no brows! And, my eyelashes are longer each time I look at them. Oddly, the upper lashes seem to be growing downward and the lower lashes are growing upwards. With any luck, in a few weeks, I will be Bambi.

One of the highlights of the past few days was the Taste of Hope benefit for City of Hope honoring an Ambassador of Hope: my good friend Zoe Mohler. It was held in Coronado and featured a delicious assortment of gourmet food and wine. Shrimp, sliders, cupcakes and the best ice cream bonbons ever! And, Kiptyn from "The Bachelorette" was the Emcee, handing out roses. All for a good cause!

Wednesday, August 24th: Fleeting moments

Today, I was reminded how fragile life can be. Not in regard to me, but in regard to the upsetting way my day began. I was meeting a new friend down in Cardiff to go for a walk and exited the house in high spirits.

As I was driving down my street, I noticed an animal in the road. Honing my gaze, I realized that it was a cat. I promptly performed an illegal u-turn and pulled up next to him. I got out of the car to assess the situation and saw that the beautiful, chocolate and black tiger-striped kitty was indeed dead. His head was lying at an awkward angle, indicating a broken neck.

Because the person who hit him hadn't bothered to stop and at least move the cat out of the street so he wouldn't be pulverized, I did so. I grabbed one of my yogitoe towels out of the trunk and gingerly lifted up the beautiful boy. He was still warm so, it hadn't been long since his life had been unceremoniously snuffed out. I moved him

235

to the grass beyond the sidewalk and left him wrapped in the pristine white blanket. I hope that his family found him. When I returned a few hours later, the blanket and kitty were gone.

So, this brings up a pet peeve of mine. I've been doing animal rescue for several years now. Often, when I speak to people wanting to adopt, they tell me that they "have to let their cats outside" for a variety of stupid reasons. No, you don't have to let the cats out: They will get hit by a car or killed by a coyote. Keep the cat indoors!

I wonder if the person who killed this cat even noticed that he'd hit something? Did he look in the rearview mirror and shrug his shoulders, oh well? Was he busy texting or talking on the phone? It breaks my heart.

Later, as I drove home on this same stretch of road, I was struck by how incredible the sky looked after sunset. It felt like I was entering a Monet landscape. Although my day had been colored with sadness for the cat I was too late to save, in that moment, I found profoundly grateful to be alive, to be able to enjoy the beauty of nature.

Jake and Oreo got extra big kisses when I walked in the door.

Thursday, August 26th: Amazing day!

Today was amazing; brimming with familiar and new faces, positive energy, interesting conversations, lots of yoga and simple happiness. The San Diego sunshine beamed down, bathing everything in a bright, soft light.

The morning began with Yoga for Cancer Recovery at lululemon. We've extended the series, so there will be two more Thursday 9 a.m. classes at the store. It is remarkable that a group of like-minded students meeting each week has become community already. I feel so blessed to be a part of something this special. When I return from Australia, we'll just move the beautiful group to a new, permanent location.

Today, I was contemplating how often I felt stuck this year. Just up against a brick wall, no progress, no options, and no prospects. Sitting in the house recovering from surgery or chemo or the ailment of the day. I had to drop so many of my regular classes and clients because of cancer.

At times, despite my best efforts, I worried about what I was going to do once treatment was done. Would I be able to make up for lost time? Were all those opportunities lost to me forever? Faith in the unknown, prayers and the unconditional love lifting me up allowed me to believe that this unchosen path of breast cancer would lead me to something new. Something powerful, true, and life-changing.

I've known for a long time that my dharma is to teach and to write on a grand scale. I remember back to 1997, when I was despondent practicing law that I would cry each morning in the shower before heading into the office. I knew then that I wanted to teach yoga and to write, reaching as many people as possible. This path is leading me to doing so in ways I could never have envisioned. My life is full of stunning opportunities. And, if that isn't a silver lining, I don't know what is.

Saturday, August 28th: Close call with Sheila

Two round-trip tickets booked for Sydney to Melbourne. A B&B selected in Melbourne and plans for an adventure road trip down the Great Ocean Road with Todd's sister Julie and her Aussie hubby Matthew. Australia is becoming a reality and less like a fantasy. We leave in less than three weeks!

Twenty-four down, 12 to go.

In terms of radiation side effects, I've yet to encounter fatigue. Perhaps because I ignored the advice of my radiation oncologist and am taking lots of antioxidants and vitamins? My energy level feels like it did pre-cancer, even though if I'm honest, I cannot remember that far back right now. The skin on my chest and right underarm, however, is angry. Red, raw, and plain livid at the radiation machine. I only have four more treatments to the large area; the remainder is to the tumor bed. Thank goodness because I think I'd have open wounds otherwise. Ouch.

My lymphedema arm has maintained for three weeks now, thank the lord! I'll continue to be extremely conservative and wear the sleeves and night sleeve until a month or so after radiation ends. Two of my new Lymphediva sleeves make me look like I've got tattoos: kind of fun.

This morning started with a potential disaster, I almost lost my wig! I went to Petco for my Rescue House volunteer session with the cats. When I arrived, I shut the door to the room and let out all of the kitties. We've got about a dozen adorable cats and kittens in there at the moment.

As I was releasing shy Jasmine from her enclosure I paused to pet her. Tyler, who lives upstairs from Jasmine, apparently got impatient. He reached out his paw and managed to pull my Sheila wig off of my head. Luckily, I grabbed it before it came all the way off and maintained my dignity. The salt-and-pepper chia pet head is not ready for public viewing yet.

The afternoon included a baby shower for a yoga instructor friend, Sara. It was great to catch up with her and a few other teachers from CorePower that I haven't seen since BC. At last, life feels like it is returning to some semblance of normalcy.

Monday, August 30th: Feeling optimistic

I'm simply simmering with optimism today. It began with teaching a lovely class, if I do say so myself, at Bindu Yoga. The energy in this beautiful little studio truly inspires. Barbara, one of my students, was kind enough to run home before class to bring me some special lotion for the radiated flesh. My chest and underarm are raw. Ouch!

I've been slathering on a variety of recommended potions, lotions and oils in what I now realize are futile attempts to prevent cooked, blistered skin. Now it looks like someone pressed a hot iron against my armpit. Yesterday I had a disquieting epiphany. When I told Meredith that I was using emu oil, she asked me how the emu oil was made. Honestly, I hadn't even considered it. Perhaps they milked the emu? Or got it from the feathers? But, I had a niggling doubt that perhaps there was a more dire explanation.

Sure enough, when I returned home, I googled emu oil and learned that they kill the emu and obtain the oil from the fat. Oh no! I'm sorry Mr. Emu. I honestly didn't realize. Back to the calendula and the aloe.

This afternoon, Robyn from City of Hope, Stacy McCarthy the yoga guru, and I met to discuss the upcoming March 5th Yoga for Hope event that we are coordinating. It is really exciting to strategize and plan

ways to create a successful, memorable inaugural event for such a worthy cause. I can't wait to confirm some details and involve yogis from all over San Diego.
I'm feeling so grateful for all the blessings in my life.

Time to slather on some more calendula aloe magic potion! Fingers crossed.

Chapter 9: September

Wednesday, September 1st: Lucky Number Eight

What a whirlwind of a day. Doctor's appointments, shopping and teaching. In that exact order.

Great news: I met with the lymphedema physical therapist for the first time in over a month. She was thrilled to see that my arm looks normal and has been maintaining for the past four weeks. The proof is in the measurements, however, and I was eager to see what the percentage decrease would be.

When we first met in June, my right arm was 14.4% larger than the left. Then, I had a horrible reaction to the heated yoga room and it ballooned up to 21.9%. Can you say elephant arm Petretti? Another month passed to reduce it down to 14% at our last meeting on July 27th.

Today, it is only an 8% difference! And, that is a 42% reduction in the size of my arm itself. Hello wrist bone! Hello elbow! Goodbye Popeye forearm! I think I may be able to wear jewelry on my right hand and wrist again after all. What a relief. I still must wear a sleeve daily and don the night sleeve each night, but I will wean off of it after radiation and hopefully only have to wear a sleeve to workout.

Anyways...

I promptly zoomed over to Nordstrom and put that newly svelte right arm and hand into action signing credit card slips. I lucked out and found some cute walking shoes for

Australia, along with some Sanctuary shorts: all on sale. I need to be prepared for my trip, right?

Next, it was Radiation Oncology for full-area treatment and new scans for the final eight treatments. Only one more "full-area" radiation tomorrow! Thank goodness as my underarm is now officially raw and blistered.

Then, Dr. L entered and drew a circle around my incision and the assistant put wire around it, which felt very strange. The assistant then stuffed me into the CT-Scanner machine again so they could photograph the wired section of boob. The final eight treatments will be directed solely to this specific tumor bed area.

In addition to the CT-Scan photos, they once again took photos with a regular camera. Snapshots of me lying on my side, with a robe half-on, wire around my magic-markered breast cancer scar. I find these very odd. All I can say is that once this blog is published as a book those photos better not surface on the Internet.

I have a reputation to uphold.

Sunday, September 5th: George Clooney and I...

have an unlikely connection. Not in any way I'd ever dreamed of, but it is unmistakable and as soon as Todd and I returned from seeing *The American*, I had to write about it.

By the way, *The American* was a disappointment. Plodding snail's pace all the way through. I'd wait for the DVD.

The epiphany that struck me during the film was that I have the exact same hair as George, except that he has about three-quarters of an inch more than me. But the salt and pepper color pattern, including full silver on the temples, dark through the center and silver in the front is identical. We even share the same little cowlick where my part will be one day soon. How did this happen? How can it be?

George is a silver fox. I am not.

I cannot wait until September 16th when I see my hairdresser and have some pretty color slapped on there. I can handle walking around with a crew cut, just not the "Cell Block 9" version.

Twelve days to Australia.

Monday, September 6th: Walking without a wig

This morning, I went for a walk wearing only a baseball cap. Well, I also had on pants, a top, shoes and socks, of course. But since I now have a little hair, albeit silver, showing in the sideburn area and at the nape of my neck, I figured what the heck?

I went to the lagoon with Kirsten, as opposed to the beach where I might actually run into someone that I know. Baby steps. It was a relief not to fuss with it. And, now that my brows and lashes are growing back, I didn't have to waste five minutes drawing on brows and liner either.

I'm thrilled to have some wasted time returned to me. Of course, it is now spent on shaving my legs that seem to be valiantly trying to make up for lost time. I'm anxious for the hair to fill in so I can go bare-headed! My fingers are crossed that my hairdresser can make it a pretty color pre-Australia.

My energy level is great and my only complaint is that the skin under my arm remains raw and weepy. Horrible.

In order to walk, I was forced to hold my hand on my hip and away from my body so I didn't exacerbate the tender skin. Very graceful. It astounds me that they proceed so far with all of these treatments despite the severity of the side effects. They saw how raw it was last week and basically just told me to deal with it. I guess I shouldn't be surprised.

Ten days to Australia...

Tuesday, September 7th: Yes I can

"There are so many people out there who will tell you that you can't. What you've got to do is turn around and say watch me." - author unknown

Life is funny: this quote arrived in my inbox this morning and it resonated strongly. Perhaps it even triggered multiple memories of me declaring just those words. And, many times I launched and I crashed back down to earth. Just as the naysayers predicted. But, many times I launched and soared. Taking risks is inherent in my being, a part of my fabric and make-up.

Life is funny: this afternoon, the folks in radiation oncology were running behind. So, I sat in the waiting room conversing with a lady waiting for her husband to be treated for oral cancer and an older gentleman being treated for I'm not quite sure what. He'd had a tumor in his lung and it was pressing on his vocal chords. Thus, he sounded strikingly like Clint Eastwood in his Dirty Harry days. He's also been going through experimental treatment over the last 18 months, had lost and regrown his hair twice, had numerous surgeries and drugs for perhaps three separate bouts of cancer.

I didn't catch his name, so I will call him Clint, in honor of the husky voice. Clint told me that when people say 'cancer' to him, he translates it to 'cure.' When people tell him his time is limited, he tells them he chooses life. He also said he still goes to the gym three times a week and does what he can because exercise plays a huge factor in staying healthy and keeping the mental attitude positive.

So, basically the Universe was giving me the exact same message twice today: once via email and once via an inspiring, strong man fighting for a cure. A cure for himself.

Interestingly, another man in the waiting room, commented to me, "You are too young to be here." And, I agreed with him. He then said, "Life isn't fair, you shouldn't be here." Again, I agreed. But if any of us in that room awaiting treatment dwell on the life isn't fair angle, we will have a tough time.

Life isn't fair. In my experience, I've found it to be true that some of us are given a lot to handle for no apparent reason. I look at my father: he's lost three of his sons, both of his daughters have had cancer, he's divorced and his only living sibling just passed away last week.

Does Rene get depressed? Maybe. But, at 86, that man is still out walking his three miles a day, he goes to play Petanque with his friends at Carderock two to three times a week, he travels back to France a few times a year to see his girlfriend and family: he is living his life. I inherited my stubborn bourrique (Corsican donkey) nature from him and I am proud of it.

Ironically, he is one of the people who consistently told me that I couldn't or shouldn't make certain choices. I ignored him. And, I'm who I am today because of that recklessness, that defiance, that fearlessness in jumping into the unknown. All my choices created who I am today, for better or for worse. I don't regret any of it. Well, maybe law school.

Thursday, September 9th: Under the weather...

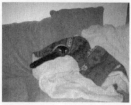

How cute is Jake burrowed under the blankets? If you look closely, you can see me there underneath them too.

So, I guess the Universe wanted me to slow down and let my radiation wound under my arm heal because Tuesday night I became very ill. Sore throat, zero ability to breathe through my nose whatsoever, dizzy, weak, nauseous. Great. The doctor took a strep culture yesterday and I'm praying that I don't have that less than two weeks prior to our trip. I was forced to cancel my clients and classes for the rest of the week.

Trapped in the house again, trying to remain immobile. In other words, I'm miserable.

I don't get sick. Well, except for this pesky little bout with cancer, I don't get sick. I hadn't had a cold in the two years before 2010.

So, I am a fan of the Neti Pot to clear out the nasal passages. The Neti Pot is a natural way to keep the sinuses and nasal passages clear and open. Sadly, I'm so congested that the Neti Pot couldn't penetrate! Nothing will flow through.

Picture this: it is 4 a.m. and I'm leaning over the sink with that bright blue Aladdin-looking pot pouring saline solution into one nostril and nothing is exiting. Then, it runs down my face as I choke and try to breathe. Repeat. How can it not work?

From all the years of yoga, I am accustomed to nostril breathing. This practice is not serving me well at the moment. Luckily, today I have the use of one-half of my left nostril so; I'm not going to suffocate.

As for the underarm: I'm not going to post a photo because some people were so disturbed by the eyebrowless-Claire photo I posted that I'm afraid I'd traumatize everyone. The doctor told me yesterday to just slather it with Aquaphor. No improvement yet and that greasy ointment is everywhere.

It seems like whenever I'm feeling excited when nearing the end of treatment, some snafu pops up. I absolutely need to be healthy because Australia is next week!! ONE week from tomorrow and I cannot be sick! Mantras of the day: Open nasal passages, open! Heal baby heal!

Saturday, September 11th: Six sleeps to Oz

Less than a week to Australia! That means that I've only got three more radiation sessions and I am finished with my cancer treatment. When will that lovely reality sink in?

I'm thrilled to report that I feel much better than I did a few days ago. The evil cold/flu bug that drove me to my knees exited stage left yesterday. My underarm radiation burn is slowly healing: a few more days to go. Three days in bed. Whew.

247

Last night, we watched the Stand Up to Cancer telethon. It was quite moving and not a little bit disturbing for me. Seeing the statistics that 207,000 people will be diagnosed with breast cancer this year and realizing that I am now one of those statistics feels strange. Part of me must be in denial. I don't know how because it only takes a glimpse in the mirror or down at my right side and I am reminded. The scars last forever, even the ones that fade on the surface. How will I feel a year from now? Five years from now?

Am I a cancer survivor? Or, is that name only applicable at 3 p.m. on Wednesday, September 15th, when my last appointment ends? Do I say that I "had" breast cancer? That I "have" breast cancer? I'm confused.

I find it rather odd that they don't have a scan when your treatment ends to declare you cancer-free. I know that they want to do a mammogram in three months and possibly every three months for the next five years? They didn't detect my cancer on my routine mammogram last September, so I am not eager to have my boob smashed in the mammogram machine so often. Imagine if I hadn't found the lump myself in January and had waited until now to go in. How far would it have spread by now?

But, I feel lucky. A new friend of mine that feels like an old friend is in the hospital. She beat cancer several years ago and now she is ill and the doctors haven't diagnosed the problem yet. She is in her 30s. When I visited her today, my gut told me she'd survive this new challenge. I know she'll beat whatever this is, even if it is cancer returning. She's too stubborn to let it take over her life. But, why does she even have to deal with it again? It seems so unfair.

248

I feel lucky to finish in three more days. Maybe I will feel done when I leave the Scripps parking lot and relinquish my Free-Parking-wristband. Or, maybe I will feel free when Todd and I are driving to LA to catch our plane. Perhaps it will register that I am finished while having High Tea in Sydney or petting a koala along the Great Ocean Road. The sooner the better!

Tuesday, September 14th: Last day treatment-eve

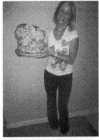

Finally, the night before the last day of cancer treatment. Coupled with the simmering excitement for this milestone is huge anticipation at leaving for Australia on Friday. Three sleeps to the adventure of a lifetime!

Not surprisingly, I am having a challenging time sleeping because I am so excited. Todd and I are zooming around in a flurry of preparations: walking shoes, trial-sized shampoo (yes shampoo people: I have an inch of hair), laundry, laying out outfits, going for increasingly longer walks to build up my stamina, choosing what to pack, and so on.

Today was full of positives: I stopped by Yoga Swami and completed the paperwork to start the weekly Yoga for Cancer Recovery classes on Thursday October 7th. It will be offered at 4 p.m. on a donation basis. I have a key and everything, so it is on!

Then, I picked up my cast from Anne Krell, the beautifully talented artist who painted it. Check it out! If I haven't written about this before, several weeks ago I was casted by the ladies from *www.keep-a-breast.org* for an upcoming Breast Cancer Awareness event being held at lululemon Carlsbad. Having someone slather plaster on my chest was an interesting experience and I must say like nothing I've ever participated in before. This group raises breast cancer awareness and education for young people using art: www.keep-a-breast.org. They are amazing.

In the middle of all of that, I taught two yoga classes, then caught up with several of my good friends on the phone and online. Later, I returned home to be surprised by Todd with a pre-vacation/end-of-treatment present.

The second-to-last radiation was a piece of cake. This is the eighth week that I've driven to Scripps every weekday. I cannot wait to turn in my hospital bracelet. I cannot wait to not enter those gates. I cannot wait to stop changing into hospital gowns on a daily basis. I cannot wait until tomorrow at 3 p.m.

Freedom.

Thursday, September 16th: Day after completion

As I ran through my itinerary for today, I automatically thought, 'Drive to Scripps' and just as swiftly, I grinned because I don't have to enter that doorway again for a few months. Today, I had more important tasks like getting a manicure/pedicure and packing for Australia. No need for any more sautéeing of my right chest.

Yesterday I was literally flying on adrenaline all day fueled by the excitement and realization that this 10-month journey is over. I. am. finished. with. cancer.

treatment. I've experienced a lot in my relatively short lifetime; it has truly been a dramatic rollercoaster ride. But, I must say that this disease or crisis or shall I just call it cancer has been the most challenging experience ever. Next chapter: blissful, exotic, million miles away vacation. This journey will be an opportunity to clear out the residue from treatment and a time for Todd and me to breathe after this incredibly difficult period.

I haven't really slept for four nights because I cannot turn off my brain. Flashes of faces keep passing in front of my eyes and I realize how many amazing people have blessed my life and supported and lifted me throughout this journey: Family, old friends, new friends, relative strangers. Todd has been a rock.

I grew much closer to some new friends and some friends faded away a bit. I know people say that you'll know who your true friends are through a crisis like this. True. What is so beautiful is that I really didn't find out anything negative: it was all positive. Instead, some people you don't expect to step up do and others who you thought would be there 24/7 aren't. My life is much richer and fuller as a result of every single one of these relationships.

And, I must say that the Oakton High School Cougars have been incredible! Shout out to everyone! Does this mean that we are all getting together over Thanksgiving in Northern Virginia? Or, does this warrant a celebratory reunion trip to Ocean City?

One sleep to Oz. I'm not sure if I will write while I am there. If not, au revoir until October.

Chapter 10: The rest...

Wednesday, October 6th: Back from Down Under

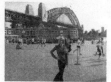

I'm baaaaaaaaaaaaaaack.

Back from what was an absolutely amazing, incredible, dare I say perfect, vacation? I'm not feeling like the brightest bulb at the moment because of the time change. We left Sydney at 3 p.m. on Sunday and arrived in Los Angeles at 10:30 a.m. the same day. "Twilight Zone". My body is baffled. I wake up at 2 a.m. ravenous and then cannot keep the eyes open at noon. Hopefully, it will balance out by the weekend.

I plan on using the next few entries to share some highlights from Oz. From seeing koalas and kangaroos on the Great Ocean Road to the "Marriage of Figaro" at the Sydney Opera House to eating and drinking enough to keep a family of four satisfied to walking for hours without getting tired. For the most part, I was able to stay present and not worry or even consider anything happening back at home. It was so healing and I really do feel "back to normal."

But my predominating theme of my hair did rear its ugly head on more than one occasion. Going through security at LAX wearing only a hat was tough because not one, but two security people asked me to remove my hat while squinting disbelievingly at my passport. I can't blame them because my hair was so short and my hairline so stark, with dyed brown hair I looked like a cross between Eminem and a teletubby. Picture a painted-on hair hat.

Who knew I should've left it salt and pepper? It isn't just that I hated feeling hideous, but that seeing that hair reminded me of the cancer. At least with a wig on, I looked more like myself.

Now, that issue is resolved because as of yesterday my hair is champagne blonde. A trainer at the gym told me that I look European. I think I look a bit like a newborn duck or chick, but I like it. A milestone day: I left the house feeling free without a wig or a hat.

After an overnight, 14-hour flight, we arrived in Sydney. The first few days, Todd and I stumbled around like a pair of drunken sailors. We were intent on staying up until at least 6 p.m. on the first day so we could adjust to the 17-hour time difference.

We stayed in an area called the Rocks, which is an incredibly charming historical part of town, right on the harbor. We could see the iconic Sydney Opera House from our hotel room window. Although those first few days are hazy in my memory, I know that I loved Sydney!

Where else can you drink a bottle of wine entitled "Ladies Who Shoot Their Lunch"? Maybe that is why those first few days were blurry?

Wednesday, October 13th Journey to a new reality

I think that I may finally be feeling like myself. What a transition!

So, I highly recommend that anyone completing cancer treatment hightail it out of town for a vacation afterwards. Somewhere incredible where you will be present and engaged, without pesky distractions like hospital gowns. I'm still riding the high from our trip to Australia. The last 10 months seem like a distant dream.

This week marks a return to a "regular" work schedule. I must admit that this is harder than I anticipated. First of all, it isn't viable for me to return to several of the classes and clients that I had to stop this year. I am mourning the communities at www.active.com and Sculpt Fusion Yoga, where I am no longer a regular fixture. The people have been fabulous and supportive and I want to be there in the capacity that I was pre-cancer, but it isn't looking feasible.

Many other doors have opened and are opening and for that, I am grateful and happy. I love starting fresh and having that excitement and anticipation of growth. Lord knows I've done it enough! And, knowing that I am different then I was in January when this all began means that I am not returning to my old life. Instead, I am launching into a new life, ready or not. Even if I did return to my exact former schedule, too much has changed.

I'm still a little shocked when I catch my reflection in the mirror and see the champagne blonde cropped hair! Who is that tough, chic creature? Talk about different. But it is so freeing to leave the house without it even occurring to me to cover my head. Fabulous.

If I focus too much on what the future holds, I feel overwhelmed and fearful. So, I remind myself to take it day by day and live in the present. My intent this week is to do that, no matter what. One of my daily intentions is to exercise for an hour each day, no matter what. I need to rebuild my physical strength and fortify my mental clarity and emotional calmness.

So far, two yoga classes and a hellish hour (seemed like 10) in Pure Barre on Monday. The two yoga classes have not alleviated the incredible soreness I am experiencing in my entire derriere yet. Ouch! I should be able to walk normally by Friday and plan on hitting Pure Barre again. Pure Barre La Costa is offering free classes to cancer survivors for the entire month of October. Generous and amazing.

Tomorrow I may make it to Zumba finally! Because now I can!

Friday, October 15th: Movin, movin, movin...

Friday afternoon. I just returned from a great Pilates session. My plan had been to take a class at Pure Barre this morning, but I didn't get any sleep last night. I thought that the hot flashes were over, but last night I alternated being drenched in sweat and shivering from the chills. Tamoxifin side effects. Please tell me that this isn't a preview of the next five years.

I achieved my goal to exercise every day. A friend commented that I must be really self-disciplined. Maybe. The reality is that I am so excited to feel healthy enough to work out, that I am eager to move daily. Now that I can go, I am grateful to do so! Pure Barre, Pilates, two yoga sessions, and my first Zumba experience.

Ahhh, Zumba with the lovely April Buck leading a full class of enthusiastic Zumba-ers. Or, is it Zumba-ettes? I am happy to report that I didn't injure myself or anyone else in the class. It was so much fun! I realized a few important truths about myself:

1. I can still grapevine with the best of them.
2. I can also still step-ball-change.
3. I have absolutely no hip action! Everyone else was rocking and rolling their hips and there I was. The hip swivels need some work! I've got no game.

What stood out the most was how everyone was laughing and smiling as we danced all over the room. Again, I feel so grateful that I am done with treatment and could fully participate. For months I've been restricted in a million different ways. Not to preach, but if you are wavering on exercising, just do it. Because you can!

Sunday, October 17th: Hair and yoga

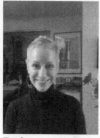

Rainy weekend. What is up with this weather in San Diego? It isn't supposed to rain in October. Ever! At least I don't have to worry about what will happen to my wig anymore! I am officially wearing my own hair: Version 2.0.

I've gotten comments from "it isn't too terrible, you can always get extensions, right?" to my personal favorite: "rocking a blonde Halle Barry." The truth, as usual, lies somewhere between these two extremes. It is just so freeing to not have to worry about what hat or hair I will don prior to leaving the house.

More importantly, the fact that my hair is now growing fast symbolizes a return to health. As it was a symbol of my sickness when I was bald, it now is a clear indicator that I am on the road to recovery. Because I feel stronger each day, I have worked out for the last seven days in a row. The only reminder is the ever-present lymphedema sleeve. My goal is to build up the activity and hold steady, then start weaning off of wearing the sleeves 24/7. I can't wait.

Yesterday, I had a breakthrough in yoga class. For the first time in several months, I was able to practice a full Vinyasa flow class without modifications. A few walls were dropped and the tears flowed. I have been craving this type of movement to release the pent-up emotions stuck in my body. Finally! I cannot describe how it feels to start feeling connected in my mind, body and heart once again.

Grateful. Ecstatic. Sad.

Emotionally, I'm a ping-pong ball. What a shocker! It just feels strange to be returning to only some of my prior teaching. Much has shifted. I know that new doorways are opening, but perhaps this gloomy weather has instilled some melancholy in my soul. I guess that is to be expected. I need to keep reminding myself not to project too far into the future.

Day by beautiful day.

Tuesday, October 19th: Saved by a fork...

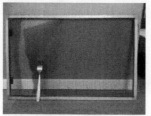

Life is returning to status quo. How do I know?

What happened this afternoon wouldn't have happened while I was going through diagnosis and treatment. The Universe or God or whatever you choose to call the powers-that-be know that this escapade would have broken me just a few short months ago. Today, I wish this had been caught on film because it must've looked hysterical.

At approximately 11:50 a.m., I exited the house to teach my 12:15 yoga class at Frogs. I had everything I needed: new yoga mix-loaded iPod, umbrella, and lunch in the form of quinoa salad from Seaside Market. I'd even brought a fork with me to eat said salad. I never bring silverware with me.

So far, so good. Well, as the door clicked shut behind me, it struck me. I didn't have my keys. No car key. No house key. Oops. No spare key stored anywhere. Todd is out of town until tomorrow night.

I was locked outside, in the rain mind you, with no way to get to class or to get back inside. Luckily, I did have my cell phone. "I'll just call the pet sitter," I thought. Well, Sally's phone just rang and rang, with no voicemail or answering machine picking up. Great.

The clock was ticking.

Next, I called Frogs and explained my embarrassing predicament to the resourceful Lori. Luckily, Franco, a yoga teacher was in the club and stepped in for me at the last minute. I was free to focus on breaking in.

Resolute, I climbed up onto our balcony on the off chance that the sliding glass door might be unlocked. It wasn't. The cats stared at me from inside, completely baffled. I exited the slippery balcony as gracefully, ahem, as I had entered it. Next, I called Todd and he suggested I break into the dining room window, which is about 4-5 feet up from ground level. Wet, muddy, leaf-covered ground level.

In vain, I struggled with the wet, cobweb-covered screen. No dice.

Returning to the front of the house, I contemplated the front door. Just me, the rain and the locked door. Wait! The fork rested on top of my pile of things on the front mat.

Then, my aha moment occurred. The fork! Prongs! The intractable screen!

I scurried back to the rear of the house. With a few sharp stabs, I'd ripped the screen apart. Next challenge: pop the stick we had in the window out so I could open it wide enough to climb inside. Completed on the third attempt.

Now that I had an opening, my next dilemma was how to get in? The window is too high for me to pull myself up. The table on the balcony called to me, so I pulled myself up again and picked up the table and dropped it off the balcony to the wet ground. With the added height from the table, I was able to maneuver myself through the window, landing with a resounding belly-flop onto the floor. Success!

Just as I landed, Sally called, offering to come over with my key and let me in. Imagine that.

Thursday, October 28th: Whirlwind week

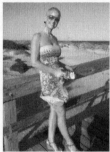

Wow, what a whirlwind since I last wrote. An amazing career opportunity dropped into my lap and I've been running around like a chicken with my head cut off to prepare all the submission requirements. It is a part-time gig and would fit in perfectly with everything else in my life. Fingers crossed!

Here's a hint: I had to order transcripts. Yes, college and law school transcripts. Really. And, of course, law schools being what they are, they won't allow you to order your transcript online. So, I had to drive up to University of San Diego Law School and walk into the Registrar's office for the first time since graduation. Can I tell you what an out-of-body experience it was to step into Warren Hall? Flashbacks flowed fast and hard. Although I maintained a shred of dignity and didn't run out of there, I'd say I moved at a fast trot to my car.

USD's campus is beautiful. I'm glad to see that my still-unpaid law school loans are keeping the gardeners in business. And, I'm sure that I saw a new wing to one of the buildings that was personally funded by my six-figure contribution.

I've frequently discussed all the risks I've chosen in my short life and my lack of regrets. Except, I do think if I had the chance for a redo, I would skip law school. Yes, skip it I would.

I'm finally settled in for a little while. It seems like we'd just gotten accustomed to home after Australia and then we flew to Savannah on Friday for my dear friend Angie's wedding. The wedding was fantastic; Angie was a beautiful bride and Darin was a proud and emotional groom. I'd say the whole experience rated as one of the most perfect weddings ever!

I'm grateful that we were able to go. Life is short, friends are dear and experiences are what matter most. And, Savannah is one of the most unique and beautiful cities I've ever seen. I tried two new foods: fried green tomatoes, which were yummy and boiled peanuts, which were not. Who thought boiling peanuts was a good idea?

Tuesday night I attended the YSC Spa Night at SK Sanctuary in La Jolla. The evening is put on by YSC and included free massages and facials, h'ors d'oevres, fabulous goodie bags and an inspiring speaker: Stefanie LaRue. Stefanie was diagnosed with Stage IV breast cancer at age 30 and told that she had nine months to live. That was five years ago. She personifies hope. I know that I felt uplifted and happy after the evening.

Now I've got to go prepare for a yoga class that I am teaching tomorrow night for Breast Cancer Awareness Month. Sculpt Fusion Yoga is hosting the class at 5:30

p.m., with all donations to benefit YSC. I'm looking forward to it!

Sunday, October 31st: Festivities, hot flashes and surprises

I'm filled with gratitude this weekend. Friends, fun and festivities.

Friday night I led a yoga class at Sculpt Fusion Yoga for Breast Cancer Awareness month. Donations went to the Young Survival Coalition, a group where I've found a great deal of support with other young women hit by cancer.

All week, I vacillated between feeling excited to teach and nostalgic for the days when I could teach there without fear. I used to teach five classes a week at SFY, but due to the chemo and radiation and lymphedema, my body betrayed me each time I stepped into the heated room. Either I'd feel dizzy and nauseated or the lymphedema flared up and my hand and arm would blow up again.

It was a great evening and wonderful opportunity to see old faces. I really miss the community. I did have a bit of a heat hangover afterwards. The class was supposed to be non-heated, but an earlier class had ended only 15 minutes prior and the heat just didn't dissipate. So, everyone got a lot sweatier than anticipated and I ended up having a hot flash kind of night...

Apparently, it takes about three months for your body to rid itself of the radiation effects. It makes sense I guess: 36 rounds of daily radiation is bound to have lingering consequences. Part of the radiation legacy is that your internal body-temperature clock doesn't work. No sleep for me. I was burning up and sweating and tossing and turning all night long. Clothes, lymphedema sleeve and even a cat or two went flying off the bed in the dark.

Teaching that class cleared up any ambiguity over whether I was ready to practice or teach in even moderate heat. No need to hurry it. I'll try again. December 15th is the three-month mark. Not unexpected, but nonetheless disappointing.

Two parties on Saturday! First stop was Lori's baby shower. She is going to be the best baby mama to little Natalie. And, Natalie is going to be a very well-dressed little girl! It was really nice to share in the celebration of new life with a lovely group of women.

Next, the fun began at 5 p.m. at Party City where Todd and I and every other Halloween procrastinator battled over masks and costumes. We emerged unscathed with a couple of ornate masks, ready for a glass of wine and a surprise birthday party for Dino. At Blanca, everyone donned masks and let's just say that the birthday boy was surprised! Friends and family traveled from as far away as Canada to share in the celebration.

A great reminder that you just never know what surprises are around the corner, right?

Wednesday, November 3ʳᵈ: Makers Mark and money

So, I've not been too consistent on the blog since my return from Australia. I'd wrestled with ending it once I set foot on the plane, but several people told me that they'd like to continue hearing my escapades as I re-enter "normal" life. Or, should I say the "new normal?" Resuming regular life is part of this journey.

To be honest, I've been stressed this week. Despite being blessed with some really awesome new opportunities,

263

despite being done with treatment, despite the love and friendship, even despite the fast pace of my hair growth, each morning when I've woken up, I've felt rough.

Part of the problem is that the hot flashes have been scorching me. We are having late summer in San Diego-- 90 degrees today!--and my inner thermostat has officially gone haywire. I must not be recovered from radiation yet and my body needs more time before I can endure heat like I did Friday night. The flashes are constantly waking me up and I am exhausted.

I did, however, apparently get some sleep last night because I had a bizarre, colorful dream. In my dream, I went to CVS to pick up my refill of Tamoxifin, the drug that gives hot flashes, and the pharmacist told me that they had a substitute for the Tamoxifin. Mind you, this is the same pharmacist I've seen way too much of at the Solana Beach CVS this year. I said, "Sure" because I just didn't care. I've wrestled with the Tamoxifin five-year-sentence, even skipping it for a few days here and there. What a rebel: ha!

At this point, the dream turned comical. She then informed me that the replacement for Tamoxifin is 50 cases of Makers Mark. For those of you, like me, who aren't familiar with Makers Mark, it's "Straight Kentucky Bourbon." I had to Google it. I am not a bourbon drinker. I'm not a liquor drinker for that matter.

Nonetheless, I acquiesced and she called an assistant to help her. The next thing I know, they are stuffing bottles of Makers Mark and stacks of $100 and $50 bills into big black duffel bags and dumping them into my shopping cart. The pharmacist has to send the assistant to get another cart because 50 cases is a lot of liquor! I'm curious to know what this all means? Perhaps they want me to just get drunk and go shopping so I won't worry about a cancer recurrence?

I am fighting to feel good day by day. Teaching, walking, spending time with friends, focusing on all the gifts that I have in my life. Sometimes I wonder why you don't wake up feeling great every day. I wonder if it is always a process, a shift to focus on the positive, a choice of how you are going to spend your day and your life. Living in the present isn't always easy, but there is no other choice if I am to remain sane.

Maybe I need to lay off the Makers Mark?

Sunday, November 7th: Fall back & Race for the Cure

Fall back: it is a bit disconcerting that this weekend symbolizes the beginning of fall, after our sun-drenched, 90-degree week. Summer in November! I love this time of year. Autumn symbolizes a time of renewal and rebirth, a time to shed the old and make room for the fresh and new. Participating in the Race for the Cure this morning seemed timely.

After sharing an excellent dinner with April and Matthew at Market last night, we made sure to turn the clocks back an hour. This was vital because we had to leave the house by 6 a.m. to meet up with the Young Survival Coalition crew.

The time was moot because I was rudely awakened at 3 a.m. by a dream that I was being roasted on a spit over an open campfire. Like a marshmallow or a weenie. Instead, when I awoke, I was drenched in sweat from these damn night sweat/hot flashes. Seriously, I am over this. When will they cease? It is the most bizarre feeling because all of a sudden the back of your neck sizzles and poof, you are cooking from the inside out. Talk about generating tapas.

Anyway, Todd and I joined up with YSC and close to 20,000 people who walked or ran in the Race for the Cure 5k. This is the first time I've ever received a medal for a race! Who cares if it was at a leisurely stroll, surrounded by groups of walkers with names like "Tits and Giggles", "Save Second Base", and the "Boobie Brigade?" I sported a YSC banner that proclaimed me a Young Survivor, with my diagnosis date and age on the back. Todd wore a bib that stated he was celebrating me and my sister Yael.

Prior to participating in the race today, I was feeling rather apprehensive. Would this be uplifting? Would it be upsetting? Would I cry? Or, would I just be slightly hung-over from one too many glasses of wine at dinner and four hours of sleep?

I'd say that this event proved to be simultaneously amazing and overwhelming. What seemed the most poignant to me were the countless groups walking in memory of a loved one. T-shirts with pictures of moms, sisters, grandmothers, and friends abounded. And, made me realize yet again that I am one of the lucky ones who officially beat cancer. With all of this positive energy, how can a cure not be imminent?

Next up this week? An interview with City of Hope tomorrow, a talk at a YSC event, Complementary Care for Cancer regarding yoga's role in recovery and then off to San Francisco to visit my BFF Megan and the world's greatest mom, Judy!

Not bad for the beginning of fall.

Wednesday, November 10th: "C" is for...

Clear!

Today I went in for my first mammogram post-cancer treatment. The radiologist said that everything looked good. I have an MRI next month, which generally shows more.

Oops, and I just realized that I still had a sticker on my boob, where they mark the incision. Just peeled off a pink sticker with a strawberry pattern on it. Wow.

So, the head of radiology, who is actually the woman who gave me two of the most painful experiences (biopsy and shooting in a radioactive isotope pre-surgery), came in to say hello. Her first comment was, "Didn't you have much longer hair before?"

Um, yes. I don't think I need to elaborate any more on that. "Did you pass sensitivity training Doctor?"

I was discussing with someone today whether I was considered "cancer-free" and my answer was "I guess so." Basically, the oncologists say that they assume the chemotherapy and radiation worked based upon the statistics. You know what they say about assumptions, right? I guess I will just begin answering with an emphatic YES that I am cancer-free until someone tells me otherwise. Think positive, right?

Oreo, my cat who was diagnosed with cancer in April, just climbed on my lap. He was given months to live and he is still hanging in there. He had to get another steroid injection on Monday and wasn't too pleased about it. But they seem to prevent him from throwing up his dinner, which is a good thing. I'm glad that he is still here.

267

Tonight I am discussing the role that yoga plays in complementary care for cancer at a Young Survival Coalition event. The evening also features Christa Orecchio on nutrition and Mark Skalr on acupuncture. I'm convinced that the combination of these three protocols played a huge role in me maintaining the amount of strength and oomph that I did. Is oomph a word?

So, perhaps I should review my notes for the talk one more time...

Friday, November 12th: Patchwork Petretti

What a week! I'm winding down from running all over town for meetings, talks, walks and teaching gigs. Time to breathe and allow my nervous system to relax. I'm flying up to San Francisco tomorrow to spend time with my BFF Megan and her amazing, wonderful mom Judy. I'm so excited.

The Complementary Care for Cancer event put on by the YSC went well. I was a little nervous, but it turned out fine. Speaking about yoga during cancer treatment and recovery should be a no-brainer, but I still cannot say, "I was diagnosed January 12th, 2010" without my voice breaking. Practice, right? Hopefully by the time that I speak in front of the 500 people at Yoga for Hope on March 5th, I will be able to do so without blubbering.

So, my gimpiness is slowly healing. My right hip flexor and hip were so out of joint that my right leg actually measured 3/4 inch shorter than the left! Can you say lopsided? Thanks to the brilliant Dan Selstead and ART therapy, I'm on the mend. I'm thrilled that I could practice yoga yesterday with few modifications.

Seriously, all I want to do is walk several days a week, practice yoga four times a week and do Pilates or Pure Barre 2-3 times. It isn't like I'm training for the Ironman.

Actually, it was quite amusing: a new Pilates client of mine and I were discussing injuries and I was commiserating. Knee: yes, I had knee surgery back in June 2007. Back issues: yes, I've got herniations and bone spurs and arthritis at L4-L5. Neck issues: Oh yes, I was in a car accident and had neck surgery and now have an artificial disc at C5-6. All of these issues of course preceded cancer and the lymphedema sleeve. She looked at me and said, "You are a mess!" I guess that is one way to look at it.

Sometimes I feel like I'm a little boat. I patch up one leak and then another one sprouts. Is this what getting older feels like? I feel like I'm hobbling around with the sore hip flexor, the lymphedema sleeve, the crazy hair, and the inability to go into the heated room because of radiation side effects. High-maintenance much?

Despite all my physical issues, I am plugging along. Nobody will stop Patchwork Petretti. My brain and my spirit want to go, go, go and this darned body is coming along, whatever it takes!

Tomorrow: yoga in the morning and then off to San Fran to spend time with two of my favorite people in the world. Life is good.

Tuesday, November 16th: Decisions, decisions...

San Francisco was lovely. Spending quality time with Megan and her mom, Judy, felt like visiting home. I believe that members of your true family are not always related through blood.

Despite enjoying myself, a few nagging side effects marred my time in San Francisco and have been weighing on me in recent weeks. This Tamoxifin. I'm into my fourth month on the drug that I believed wasn't affecting me too badly, except for the hot flashes. I thought they were dissipating, but actually they are not. One second I'm comfortable, the next I am sweating like a hooker in church. How bad is that cliché? Hee hee.

In addition to the pesky 20-degree internal thermometer swings, I've continued to feel heavy, almost leaden when I wake up in the morning. Instead of springing out of bed ready to embrace the day, I have to very consciously psyche myself up. Once the day is in full-swing, however, I feel engaged in whatever I am doing.

From what I understand, this is a chemical reaction from the Tamoxifin and perhaps some leftover effects from chemo and radiation. I don't like it. I don't like it one bit. I'm happy. Darn it. Seriously, everything is going very well for me. I've gone on several amazing trips, I am living and loving the present, my days are filled with loving caring people, and I've got exciting plans for the immediate future in both the work and play arenas. In other words, there is no reason for me to feel depressed.

I consulted with the YSC group to see if others have felt this way. Oh yes. I have not lost that last marble! Reports of hot flashes, mood swings, depression, anger, weight gain, and insomnia across the board. It is comforting to know I am not alone!

So, again we come to the debate of quality of life vs. staying on the medication. Kind of where I was when I wanted to stop after four rounds of chemotherapy. Well, one woman's story has convinced me to stay on the Tamoxifin for now. She chose to stop it and four years later, the cancer returned, metastasizing in her bones and liver. They are actually now treating her, ironically, with the Tamoxifin and it is working.

So, I guess I'll continue to be a sweaty, despondent beast for the next four years, eight months.

When I consulted with my doctor, she prescribed Effexor because she says it will help with the hot flashes and the heavy head. More pills. I'm leery of introducing another drug into my system. I really don't want to take anything. But, I am tempted to try it for a few weeks and see if it helps. I'm also exploring the herb/acupuncture route. I'm increasing my yoga and exercise each day. It all has to help, right?

Just the other day, we were laughing at some of the pharmaceutical commercials on television. Idyllic scenes, depicting couples and puppies frolicking in fields filled with butterflies lounging on plump flowers with a soothing voiceover reading side effects like those listed below.

The Effexor side effects:

THE GOOD: Headache, drowsiness, dizziness, nausea, weakness, dry mouth, constipation, loss of appetite, weight loss (the only two positives in the lot), blurred vision, tiredness, nervousness, trouble sleeping, sweating, yawning. May increase blood pressure...

THE BAD: Call your doctor about severe pounding headache, unusual or severe mental/mood changes, shakiness, decreased interest in sex, changes in sexual ability, difficulty urinating....stomach/abdominal pain, chest pain, persistent cough, shortness of breath, bloody/black/tarry stools, vomit that looks like coffee grounds, easy bruising/bleeding, fast/irregular pounding heartbeat, muscle weakness/cramps, yellowing eyes/skin, dark urine, seizures, unusual tiredness...

THE UGLY: If that isn't enough for you, you may get "Serotonin Syndrome" featuring hallucinations, fainting, restlessness, loss of coordination, severe dizziness, unexplained fever, nausea/vomiting/diarrhea, and twitchy muscles. Men may get a four-hour erection. Really.

Decisions, decisions.

Thursday, November 18th: Yoga to the rescue again!

Today, I was reminded once again of the power of practice. I attended a lovely Vinyasa class and felt so calm and peaceful afterwards. It feels wonderful to be able to practice the style of yoga that I love again. What a gift. Stepping onto the mat feeling off and exiting it feeling on. I swear it's like a recalibration from the inside out. Wake up, yoga, rest, repeat.

I also saw Lois, my fabulous acupuncturist, to discuss using acupuncture and TCM, traditional Chinese medicine, to deal with the hot flashes and the head. I feel very confident in her skills and the strength of natural remedies. The alternative isn't viable. I'll tell you why.

There is an excellent reason that I didn't blog yesterday. My pupils were enormous, chills shot up and down my spine and arms, my reaction time was a half-beat behind everyone else's and I just felt weird. Driving felt like I was a player in a video game. Why? I succumbed in a moment of desperation to Effexor on Tuesday and Wednesday. Let's just say that it was a disaster. Medicine affects me strongly and although this was a minimal dosage, it made me totally crazy. I'd rather wake up melancholy and break into spontaneous sweat-fests several times a day then feel that way for an hour.

Maybe I should hang a poster saying "Don't worry, be happy" on the ceiling above my bed so it is the first thing I see in the morning. Life is beautiful and precious and every single minute counts. Nobody knows how long we've got on this earth and I'm going to enjoy my time, sweaty or not.

Monday, November 29th: Day by day

My, oh my, the blog entries have been few and far between this month! I guess now that I'm running around like a chicken with my head cut off, I've not been as diligent in committing words to paper. I'm not even sure where to begin.

Thanksgiving in Virginia was lovely. Before flying home, I was apprehensive about the trip. I hadn't seen any family and friends since going through treatment and part of me didn't feel up to talking about treatment and didn't feel like explaining my punk rock hairdo. Of course, being with my family felt very positive and I was happy to see everyone's relief at me looking healthy. After a few glasses of wine, everyone was telling me that I should keep my hair short because I looked like a model. Keep on drinking people! It isn't terrible, but it feels like a charade. Let's just say I am continuing to grow it as fast as I can!

The most exciting news is that I received confirmation that my new part-time professional endeavor will start in January. I've been hired as an assistant professor at MiraCosta College in Cardiff. What will I be teaching you ask? I'll be teaching in the Kinesiology/Health Department for the Yoga Certification program. I've always enjoyed teacher training and this will be an

273

awesome venue. I cannot wait! This will round out my schedule very nicely.

My strength and flexibility continues to grow each day. I'm consistently practicing yoga and with each class I am able to do more and more of the Vinyasa flow that I love. One of these days I anticipate feeling completely at home in my body again. I'm definitely receiving daily lessons in patience, acceptance and humility.

Life is good.

Wednesday, December 1st: An emotional week

Throughout my treatment, one of my persistent themes seemed to be that I felt stagnant, that life was passing me by, that everyone and everything else was moving forward and I was stuck in cancer treatment limbo.

Well, that phase is most definitely over.

Now, I'm holding on tight as life is speeding along at an incredible rate. The blessings, the gifts, the amazing people that I am meeting, the joy that I am feeling are slightly overwhelming. All in a good way, but wow!

I am really excited about the new job at MiraCosta College starting next month. My hefty HR packet arrived, which makes it all seem very official. I'll be working with an awesome group of people, getting paid to do what I love. I've missed being an active part of a yoga teacher training program and am really looking forward to it. Time to dive deep!

Also, I've been blogging less because I've been focused on crafting a query letter to find a literary agent. I'm adapting this blog into a book. Based on all of the feedback that I have received, I believe that I can really help others with my story. So, I've been researching agents and starting the process of getting published. Fingers crossed!

This week has been very emotional. World AIDS Day struck me quite hard as I paused to remember my brother Paul, who died at age 27 and my brother Andre who died at age 33 from this disease. Although it has been 20-plus years now, it still feels like yesterday. I suppose you never really recover from that type of loss, do you? Tragic. Everything seems to be striking me powerfully. I've shed more tears in the last few weeks then I have in the last six months. Release much?

On that note, my friend Tracy took me to the most magical, fabulous yoga class ever. We went to the Yinki class at Soul of Yoga on Thursday night. We were in Pigeon for six minutes on each side and the teacher was also performing Reiki healing. I've been battling a hip-flexor issue in my right hip forever. After that class, I felt like I've been healed. It is nothing short of miraculous. I'm so excited at this discovery!

My body finally is starting to feel like MY body again. I took some great classes this week and some shifts are occurring. Finally. Patience is not my greatest virtue (ahem) and it has been a challenge this year to contend with all the delays in returning to a regular yoga and Pilates practice. I feel that I've crossed the line into truly feeling at home in my body again. Unifying the physical body with the emotional and mental bodies at last.

On a humorous note, I learned that my body is on the lululemon website! They used some of my ambassador photos. If you go to the site, there I am under Jackets and Pants. What is the funny part? My head is cut off. I don't know whether I should feel offended or flattered? I think I'll just stick with amused.

Monday, December 13th: Insomnia, please go away

It is 1 a.m. Sunday night and I am wide awake. When will the insomnia stop plaguing me? I fell asleep normally, but woke up about 45 minutes ago. Sleep eludes me. Instead of suffering in bed, tossing and turning, I'll write.

Why am I awake? Let's see: my lymphedema is flaring up again and the giant oven-mitt night sleeve squeezes my arm like a python preparing dinner. When I remove it to type on the computer, the grooves on my arm are deep. In fact, this sleeve has woken me up numerous nights simply from the discomfort. I guess that means it is working?

Next, the hot flashes are slamming me again. I think it is time to see Lois again for some acupuncture. As I write, my face feels suffused with heat.

And tomorrow, or should I say today, I've got my first MRI check-up post-treatment. We did the mammogram a few weeks back and it was declared clear. Well, last September my mammogram was normal and I found the tumor four months later. Not exactly reassuring.

In February, the MRI was one of a myriad of tests that really sucked. Horrible. They put an IV in my arm with dye which was excruciating and then stuffed me face down into the MRI machine. I do not relish repeating the experience.

So, I guess the combination of these three concerns is keeping my brain active despite the exhaustion of my mind and body.

Life continues to fly at a pace that I can barely handle. There is so much to do! All positive! I continue to remind myself to breathe. Pause and breathe. I must be more stressed than I realized.

Between preparing the syllabus and course outline for the spring semester at MiraCosta, arranging and attending meetings for the upcoming Yoga for Hope event, sending out query letters to agents for my proposed book, being interviewed for *Vision Magazine*, setting up a meeting with a videographer to discuss filming a DVD for Yoga for cancer recovery, preparing for Christmas, and continuing to build my yoga practice and physical activity back up to pre-cancer levels and oh yes, teaching. I'm riding the magic carpet ride!

Micaela and Todd from EpicPhotoJournalism took some amazing photos of me for the Yoga for Hope event... A symbol of rebirth and healing.

I am looking forward to a lull in the activity to reflect on all the changes for 2010. Some powerful transitions and transformations this year. I feel blessed to feel as good as I do and to have so many amazing people in my life.

Wednesday, December 29th: Musings on 2010

For last year's words belong to last year's language. And next year's words await another voice. And to make an end is to make a beginning. -- T.S. Eliot

As 2010 concludes, I must admit that I feel a great deal of pressure to create a few pithy blog entries. Lovely passages that sum up this rollercoaster of a year. Lovely passages thanking all the beautiful people in my life without whom I wouldn't have survived. Lovely passages reflecting in a tidy manner all that I am thankful for. Lovely passages listing out all that I have learned. Lovely passages wrapping up this year-long journey in a beautifully bow.

Wouldn't that be lovely?

Instead, I have to say that December has been scattered, at best. Talk about changes. Endings. Beginnings. I haven't sat down and truly reflected on everything that transpired this year, both cancer and non-cancer related. Or, is everything somehow cancer related because the bulk of my time was spent fighting it?

Last December, I had a reading from a Psychic/Tarot reader who told me that I would receive all I wanted in this lifetime: love, success in my chosen endeavors, passion, security, but at a price. She said that my life was tinged with the bittersweet and that as long as I could accept the bitter with the sweet, I would be fine. So, in reviewing 2010, let's see if that holds up.

It is true that you should never give up hope because you never know what is just around the corner. Who could have predicted on January 1st where I would be today?

Or, on January 12th, when I was formally diagnosed with cancer?

One of my dreams is to become a successful author: I now have a full manuscript and am in the process of submitting it for publication. What was the price? Cancer. It may take me a while to get it published, but I've proven to myself that I can write daily and be disciplined. Finishing my romance novel is next.

My passion is sharing the gift of yoga. Yoga truly helped me make it through this year and to be able to share that with others living with cancer is rewarding.

I have bonded with some amazing people and am thrilled at the richness and depth of the burgeoning relationships. What was the price? Letting go of other relationships that did not withstand the cancer. I know that people often come into your life for a period of time and then move on and that is okay. I am still very sad at some of the losses, but am choosing to accept and let go. My family and true friends have been amazing and I am not yet able to articulate all I am feeling in that regard.

Todd stood by me throughout this most challenging of years and really showed me how real our love is. We are enjoying re-establishing the new normal. I don't know how you ever really thank someone for all the love and selfless devotion it takes to be the partner of someone in treatment for cancer. I guess by healing and moving on? Or, a Rolex?

I just cannot believe that it has been almost a year. Wow. I am not going to say that I am a better person for having cancer because I don't think that I am. It has definitely changed my path and deepened my purpose in helping and healing. But at the end of the day, I am the same

Claire who loves the people in her life, the same Claire that is the little old cat lady in training, the same Claire who loves teaching, the same Claire who likes to rock out to Guns N Roses, the same Claire who yells at all the incompetent drivers, the same Claire that loves bread, cheese, wine and chocolate.

Same old Claire: now if the hair would just grow faster!

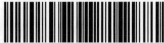

Made in the USA
Charleston, SC
30 July 2014